Keeping Your Heart in Rhythm

The Lifestyle Enhancement Institute Contributory Series

Laurie S. Abelbeck, J.D. and Alfred F. Lynch, M.B.A., Contributing Editors

Never Grow Old: Aging Healthfully Into Your Hundreds and Beyond (presently being written)

Keeping Your Mind Sharp at Any Age (presently being written)

Generations, Planning Your Legacy

Legacy: Plan, Protect and Preserve Your Estate

Ways and Means: Maximizing the Value of Your Retirement Savings

Keeping Your Heart in Rhythm

✦

The Seven Natural & Safe Ways to Protect Against Irregular Heartbeats…

Without Expensive Drugs, Surgery and other Invasive Procedures

A Special Edition

Stuart B. Kalb, J.D., LL.M.

Plus Special Bonus **Section: Natural & Safe Ways to Keep Your Heart in Perfect Health-***Without Drugs, Surgery or Other Invasive Procedures*

iUniverse, Inc.

New York Lincoln Shanghai

Keeping Your Heart in Rhythm
The Seven Natural & Safe Ways to Protect Against Irregular Heartbeats...

iUniverse books may be ordered through booksellers or by contacting:

iUniverse
2021 Pine Lake Road, Suite 100
Lincoln, NE 68512
www.iuniverse.com
1-800-Authors (1-800-288-4677)

ISBN-13: 978-0-595-36450-3 (pbk)
ISBN-13: 978-0-595-81203-5 (cloth)
ISBN-13: 978-0-595-80882-3 (ebk)
ISBN-10: 0-595-36450-0 (pbk)
ISBN-10: 0-595-81203-1 (cloth)
ISBN-10: 0-595-80882-4 (ebk)

Printed in the United States of America

DISCLAIMER

The author, the editor and the publisher are not engaging or attempting to engage in medical advice or similar professional services. The author is not a medical doctor. The author cannot diagnose or treat anyone's medical conditions. Also, the author is not intending to prescribe the use or the discontinuance of any medication as a form of treatment without the advice of an attending physician, either directly or indirectly.

You are advised that anything that you do in connection with the suggestions and opinions outlined in this book should be done under the supervision of a licensed medical doctor, and if you don't you are doing things at your own risk. This book is being written for educational purposes only and the views, opinions and statements are not intended to be an attempt to prescribe any medical treatment. The information is solely the author's opinion, unless otherwise stated, based upon the information (scores of reports, books, journals, and articles read and analyzed by the author) currently available. It is the intent of the author is to offer information on the importance of keeping your heart healthy and in good rhythm and to inform you of how environmental factors, lifestyle and some of the things you place in your body tend to cause irregularities within, or damage to, your cardiovascular system.

This book is not intended as a replacement for sound medical advice from a physician. In fact, sharing the information contained in this book with your attending physician is highly desirable.

Although the issues covered in the book have been checked and validated with sources believed to be reliable, some material may be further affected by additional discoveries since the manuscript for this book was completed. For that reason, the accuracy and completeness of such information and the opinions based thereon are not guaranteed. In addition, since everyone reading this book has genetic and metabolic differences, the strategies outlined in this book may not be suitable for every individual.

Managing Editors: Laurie S. Peck, J. D. and Alfred F. Lynch, M.B.A.

Contents

Part II   Keeping Your Heart Healthy – Period

Forward

During the final years of my father's life, I frequently visited him in an assisted living facility in Florida. I was always fascinated with the one-dimensional preoccupation with a topic of conversation amongst the residents of the facility – notably, what ails them. The whole remainder of their lives was focused on their problematical health and in many cases their heart health. Similarly, in visiting with elderly estate planning clients in my practice I have observed the same common topic of conversation, notably, a preoccupation with their physical ailments and the drugs that they are reliant upon.

There is an overwhelming general sense of inevitability in connection with their fate – that they will get old, they will get ill (in one or more ways) and they will have to rely on the mainstream medical community and prescription drugs to keep them alive. And, as to people who are healthier and younger, there is also a common theme, notably a philosophy that a lack of pain and discomfort is the equivalent of a lack of health problems. Sure, people go to doctors to address a problem or to see if a problem exists, but what do most people really do to prevent health problems from occurring in the first place? And, to what extent do most people actually challenge the fact that the majority of foods, drinks or other consumables (that are not deemed to be illegal) provided by our modern food distribution system are simply non-nutritious, downright unhealthy, and/or even toxic? Is it possible that such foods, drinks and other consumables got that way as a result of the manner in which they were created, treated, prepared, processed and/or packaged?

There is little knowledge or even concern about the prevention of illnesses and diseases by the average American consumer. This is because, as you will read, there is not much profit for American business (and actually, our economy as a whole) in making the American public aware of time-tested preventative techniques that could have the effect of eliminating the need to purchase hundreds of billions of dollars of healthcare goods and services. After all, if we are healthy, doesn't it necessarily follow that we will go to the doctor and other medical professionals less, the hospital less, and use drugs less, if at all. Insurance companies will charge less and make less money. We will not buy and eat as much food, particularly the very addictive salted, spicy, fried and high-carb foods that are otherwise so tasty, yet so unhealthy – because we don't need them.

I believe that many of our prescription and non-prescription drugs are unneeded and even dangerous; our doctors and hospitals cause (in addition to preventing) tens of thousands of deaths per year; many life saving, inexpensive, natural procedures, foods, herbs and supplements are being suppressed; our Government continues to condone the consumption of toxic or extremely hazardous, as well as highly addictive, consumables like cigarettes, aspartame, sugars, excessive salt usage, simple carbohydrates, and the like. And, why? The answer is plain as day – profits! Big business makes more money by providing foodstuffs that taste good, provide instant pleasure and cause us to physiologically crave them again and again. Our drug companies and healthcare providers are motivated by profits, because it's something they are required to do as an organization and it is a goal that will ultimately enrich those individuals who run these organizations. Terms such as "prevention, causation, natural (not to mention inexpensive) cures, elimination of disease" are essentially taboo because it reduces and can even eliminate profitability of these organizations. After all, as long as millions of people are sick, billions of dollars in profit can be made each year.

After all, if you are healthy, would you spend your money on expensive prescription drugs and medical treatments? Hardly. Essentially, the healthcare providers (doctors, hospitals, drug companies, non-profit money raising trade organizations, foundations, and lobbyists) would be out of profits and out of business.

And, our Government is involved in this hypocrisy as well. It must continually cope with the dual pressure of generating tax revenues and reducing expenditures. And, to a large degree, this latter objective would necessarily suggest that it is in our Government's best interests to suppress movements and methods to prolong the lifespan of its populace. To be sure, look at our federal food and drug laws, which state that the only thing that can cure a disease is a drug. Natural remedies cannot and any claim to that effect is illegal. If anyone or any entity ventured to try to claim such a natural remedy did cure a disease, that person or entity would have to spend a fortune (several hundred million dollars) to get the natural cure approved as a drug and then expect to recoup its costs through sales. The "rub" is that natural remedies cannot be patented, which has always been the key to the drug companies' financial success. If they cannot be patented, competition would be keen and the price would be very inexpensive and it would not be worth it from the standpoint of profitability.

So, is our healthcare system working? Well, the answer depends upon your perspective. If you are a physician or hospital where your profits are reliant upon people curing illnesses and injuries, the system is doing just fine. If you are a pharmaceutical company where your profits are reliant upon the populace's having plenty of illnesses and diseases, it is a very successful system. If you are an executive of a non-profit healthcare trade organization or foundation where your job and your organization's existence depend upon people continuing to have illnesses from the disease you are raising money for, then it has been a very successful system as well. After all, we seem to have more cancer, diabetes, heart disease, arthritis, allergies, herpes, multiple sclerosis, muscular dystrophy, migraines, colds and flu, yeast infections, prostate problems, depression, insomnia, stomach problems, attention deficit disorders, sexual dysfunction, and infertility, amongst many other ailments, than at any time in our country's history. And, we seem to be spending more money and taking more prescription drugs than at any time in our country's history.

But, if you are not one of the millions of Americans whose livelihood comes from the healthcare industry, do you really believe that it is not easy to conclude that the American healthcare system is nothing more than a huge failure in terms of preventing what ails you? Americans seem to have been brainwashed into believing that you must get ill, you must get old and infirm and you must rely upon more medical treatment and more diagnostic testing (to discover more medical problems), as well as more costly surgery, invasive medical procedures and prescription drugs throughout your lives.

So, just ask yourself, can you really rely on your hospitals, your doctors, your drug and even your food suppliers and your own Government to develop substantive, permanent, and economical ways to prevent illness as well as truly and totally cure disease? Is there any incentive for the healthcare industry to have people free from disease? And, is there any system presently in place to reverse this perpetual profit syndrome of big business and big Government at the expense of your own health and well-being?

If you are a retiree, a baby boomer about to hit retirement age, or someone 30 or 40 something, you need to have a wake up call. That is, you are living longer than ever before and healthcare costs are getting get higher than ever before. And, it is a known fact that if you are the average American, you are very inadequately prepared for the financial rigors of your retirement years from a financial standpoint. And, at the zenith of this problem are healthcare costs. Medicare funding problems in the coming decades can only make the crisis get worse. Thus, it behooves all Americans to find substantive ways to simply avoid the healthcare system in their retirement years at all costs – literally! In fact, there has never been a greater need for you to engage in comprehensive strategies to prevent illness and disease so that you can greatly minimize subjecting yourself to the increasingly expensive mainstream healthcare system – a system that can devastate your accumulated assets. And, heart disease, being our nation's number one killer and disabling illness, should be at the absolute top of your list in terms of prevention techniques.

◆   ◆   ◆

About 25 years ago I was working as a senior trial attorney for the U.S. Treasury Department (Office of Chief Counsel) based in Jacksonville, Florida. I had tried a very important tax shelter case several weeks earlier and was spending some time at home writing a brief of the facts, law and analysis of the case. Now, of course, I was 30 years old at the time and there was really nothing that had gone wrong with me physically other than basic illnesses, such as colds and flu from time to time. I had never been in the hospital and had never had surgery. My physicals were always near perfect, fortunately.

I was working feverishly on the brief one morning and decided to pull an electrical plug out of a wall socket to replace it with another lighting fixture. Well, as fate would have it, when I bent over to pull out the plug, I felt a twinge in my lower back that went away briefly, but became more painful each hour as the day wore on. My right thigh was becoming numb and I had difficulty straightening up. Later that afternoon, it got so bad that when I went to the doctor, I had to literally crawl into the doctor's office.

Yes, after 30 years, my body had finally broken down and had to be fixed by the mainstream medical community. Now, back diagnosis and treatment were a lot less sophisticated in 1980 than it is today, so I underwent a series of tests and procedures to correct the situation. First, there was traction in the hospital for four days. Then there was an uncomfortable procedure called a "*mylegram*", involving the injection of radioactive dye in my spine along with taking a bunch of pictures on a cold, hard x-ray table. After the test was over, I had to spend many hours of recovery lying on my back in a certain position; otherwise the dye could cause problems. This position of lying on my back caused additional problems with urination, which was probably the most memorable part of that dreadful experience. The test ultimately showed that I had a herniated disk that most likely required surgery, but the neurosurgeon decided to try a couple of other measures first, which of course did not work. So, the only remedy left to try was surgery, which at the time was far from a perfect science.

But, while recuperating from the mylegram at the hospital, I remembered seeing a commercial on TV for an exercise type of machine that allowed me to hang upside down (with boots that wrap around your ankles with a hook to hang on a bar upside down) to relieve the pressure on my spine that gravity had been causing all my life. It made sense to me – just reverse the process that caused my back injury in the first place. Why go through surgery with all the costs and attendant risks.

So, I called my doctors and I was able to convince one of them to write me a prescription for this upside down anti-gravity machine (it was called inversion therapy at the time). Fortunately, my insurance company actually reimbursed me for the cost, and I started immediately after I received the machine. I began by simply hanging upside down and did several stretching and torso loosening exercises. I eventually was able to do an upside down sit up, and was I proud. Well, to make a long story short, I eventually cured myself – hanging upside down doing upside down stretches and sit-ups (I actually progressed to the point where I was accomplishing 50 sit-ups). Each morning I would get up and turn on the rather motivational soundtrack from the old "Rocky" movies and go to town, so to speak.

This was my first bout with my body breaking down and a realization that I was taking it for granted. It also clued me in on many of the flaws in our healthcare system at the time and how overrated it was. In short, I realized that I had to be responsible for, and take control of, my healing. Did this natural non-drug, non-surgical procedure (inversion therapy) correct my herniated disk problem? In my case and in my opinion, it unequivocally did. Did all the procedures recommended (short of risky surgery) by the mainstream medical community work? No they did not – for me.

The point of this story is that you simply must be proactive in taking control of your own wellness destiny. After all, the days of the family doctor being a true healer are over. The days where your physician coming to see you at your residence when you are sick are over. The days of true personal care and caring by health care professionals are over. You are now in an era (in terms of healthcare) where the predominant objective is profits as compared with healing, where true curing takes a back seat to risk management to prevent lawsuits, and where the dispensation of drugs totally dominates the pursuance of alternative remedies.

◆   ◆   ◆

Physicians (primarily cardiologists) are very good at studying the cardiovascular system, knowing how it works and why it stops working. They are also very good at diagnosing most heart ailments when they come about, and are very good at treating these conditions, and in some cases reversing them. Whether its hypertension (high blood pressure), angina, heart attack, congestive heart failure, stroke, carotid artery disease, or peripheral vascular disease, just to name a few, the mainstream medical community is relatively knowledgeable.

Shockingly, the medical profession unfortunately really does not specifically know what causes these benign arrhythmias and palpitations. And, it certainly does not know how to safely treat the condition, as well as many heart ailments, without the dispensation of strong drugs and the concomitant, potentially dangerous side effects of such drugs. You know this because your doctor cannot do anything else for you or someone you care about who is burdened with heart problems, inclusive of benign arrhythmias.

Sadly, many doctors are, to a limited extent, the glorified sales people for the drug companies and are the only parties that can get you drugs. It is in their best interests to continue to promote and impose drugs on their patients, mainly because it is what they have been trained to do in medical schools. It is what causes patients to keep coming back to them – notably, to get more and more drugs. And, as an added bonus for the drug companies, many of the drugs they manufacture have side effects, which must be treated or dealt with in some manner. And, it's amazing how the drug companies just seem to have other drugs (very expensive drugs) for those side effects as well. The whole process is a fascinating, never-ending profit machine, all at the expense of the American consumer and Government entitlement programs.

Why does some other symptom or problem start to develop when you take a particular drug to reduce or eliminate a symptom of an illness or disease? Why is it that so many people have so many drugs? Is it possible that the more drugs people take, the sicker they get, mainly because all drugs have negative side effects? One must wonder if the drugs are needed to merely suppress symptoms and counteract the side effects of other drugs rather than address the cause. Indeed, one could argue that prescription and non-prescription drugs are the cause of many diseases and illnesses.

The other sad part is that the drug companies are spending more and more money (in the hundreds of millions of dollars) on advertising and creating the "brainwashing" marketing propaganda that encourages the focus on medicines – particularly heart medicines. Alternative remedies and treatments are simply not in the best interests of the drug companies. The situation has gotten to the point where the drug companies are so portentous and overbearing, they now psychologically train you (through the placement of billions of dollars in media advertisements) to be the party that wants, and even needs, the drugs, rather than the doctor telling you what you need. The drug companies produce commercials with highly paid actors who are directed to portray beautiful, happy people whose lives are so much better with the drug. The commercials tell you about the wonderful pleasure the drug provides; and if you are part of that segment of the American public affected by the malady you are supposed to go run out and get the drugs you just saw on the commercial. Of course, this will tend to keep the vicious cycle of drug use going, that is, train the American consumer (i) to want the drugs rather than making the decision rest solely at the physician level and (ii) to believe there is no other safe alternative. Their advertising dollars focus on the primary human natural urge, as well as frailty – succumbing to whatever will cause more instantaneous pleasure versus future potentially painful consequences and negative side effects.

As reported in the Journal of the American Medical Association and the Washington Post on April 27, 2005, a recent study only fueled the fire of controversy surrounding the estimated $4 billion spent each year by the drug industry on direct-to-consumer advertising. The study involved sending actors pretending to be patients complaining of symptoms of stress and fatigue into 152 doctors' offices to see whether they would be given prescriptions. (The physicians had previously consented to participate but were not told when they would be tested.) Researchers found that "patients" were five times as likely to walk out of doctors' offices with a prescription when they mentioned seeing an ad for the heavily promoted antidepressant Paxil. Critics contend that the results of a study such as this one illustrate the indiscriminate approach to health product promotion that is motivated by the pharmaceutical industry's greed for profits.

To be sure, just think about what would happen if other industries operated, and were treated by the federal government, like the pharmaceutical industry. A satirical and rather amusing look at this hypothetical situation was portrayed in the July 22, 2005 edition of News Target, an online periodical. Just think – since most prescription drugs are a 30,000 markup over cost, a car would cost a mere $4 million. But, if you bought the same car in another country like Mexico or Canada, the price would be just $5,000. Automaker would justify this price by saying they needed the money to fund research and development, but in reality, most of their research would be funded by taxpayer dollars through government grants and university research centers. Meanwhile, automakers would be lobbying Congress to prohibit motorcycles, bicycles and forms of public transportation, just as the drug companies attempt to do with herbs and natural nutritional supplements. And, if you drove a Toyota purchased in another country, you would be arrested since auto imports would be banned. And, the analogy gets even more bizarre as auto dealers would be bribed with money, free vacations, free food, and free cars by automobile sales representatives to push certain cars.

In terms of safety, our federal government would focus more on the dangers of bicycles and cars with no seatbelts, airbags, crumple zones, or other safety systems would be declared perfectly safe. Driver's education programs would be terminated nationwide, and Americans would be encouraged to buy new cars rather than repair damaged ones or avoid accidents in the first place. Safety tests revealing that cars are dangerous would be hidden, and scientists who produced such results would be prevented from ever conducting car safety tests ever again. After being sued by customers injured in the automobiles with no safety systems, automakers would further lobby Congress to pass laws protecting car companies against class-action lawsuits. Any federally mandated warnings about car safety problems would be printed in small type on a tiny label hidden under the driver's seat.

In terms of advertising, we would see pictures of cheerful, fit, and energetic drivers, but the cars would break down constantly and fail to perform as represented. The cars would be sold to you with extra features like a sunroof, air conditioning, or a navigational system, but when the car arrived none of these features would be included, just as drug companies exaggerate the "multiple health benefits" of their products. Auto companies would heavily promote new models each year, which would be no different from the ones they were selling 30 years ago. The auto companies would invent reasons for you to buy many cars, just like the drug companies try to invent new, sometimes even fictitious, diseases (such as female sexual dysfunction (FSD), general anxiety disorder (GAD) and others) and they try to sell you drugs to treat those perceived afflictions. Essentially, the drug companies want to define as many people as they can as diseased, and then convince each one of them that they need a lifetime of drugs to manage such diseases.

All of this is as fascinating as it is irreverent, and there is certainly a modicum of logic surrounding this analogy.

◆   ◆   ◆

There are four very important thoughts that can be gleaned over a lifetime in connection with your heart health:

First, you must be very proactive in terms of controlling the quality of your health. You cannot rely on the institutions you have come to trust (like the healthcare industry, the food distribution industry, and even our own government to a certain degree) to look out for your best interests from the standpoint of your health and well-being. There are other hidden and not so hidden agendas of these institutions and industries, which agendas have a demonstrably negative impact on your health and well-being.

Second, the harm that you necessarily do to your cardiovascular system (and your body as a whole) at an earlier point in your lifetime frequently does not manifest itself (in terms of physical deterioration, debilitating illness or injury and pain) until a much later point in your lifetime. Often, it is too late to reverse the ailment when it occurs. This is true whether the harm is voluntary or involuntary or caused by eating the wrong foods, too much alcohol, excessive drug use, too much sun or too much smoking, and so forth.

Third, you have to work harder and harder at keeping your body in shape as you get older, particularly as to your heart health. Your heart and your body break down, much like your car breaks down over time. As your car gets older it needs more care (and, of course, the more care you give it throughout its life, the greater the chance it will last a long time). Similarly, as you get older your heart needs more care. Where the analogy "breaks down" so to speak, is that when your car is falling apart, you can easily get another one – many times a new one. However, with your heart you do not have that luxury. The best you can expect is a used one (via heart transplantation) at a cost of $200-$300 thousand, and that is if you can find one let alone having the money to pay for it.

Fourth, you cannot totally rely on mainstream medical professionals to keep you healthy. They may be able to treat problems and even cure them in certain cases. But as far as prevention in concerned, I submit to you that keeping you in tip top shape from a preventative standpoint is grossly lacking from mainstream medical professionals.

Having said all that, one of the main reasons for a lack of pro-activity is a lack of knowledge about the subject matter. Part I of the book you are about to read primarily focuses on a type of healthcare concern that also commands that you are proactive in preventing or suppressing. It is a very real heart ailment that is present in millions of people all over the world – notably, benign heart palpitations and arrhythmias. In other words, they are heartbeat irregularities that do not result from any diagnosed heart ailment. And, in most cases the condition seems to manifest itself in normal, healthy, active people. We will compare these arrhythmias with other more serious arrhythmias that are prevalent in people with heart disease. This book is designed to give you a specific, definitive, and easy-to-understand plan of attack that is designed to prevent, demonstrably reduce and/or even eliminate irregular heartbeats,

And, it does not stop there. Part II of the book also has an entire bonus section on keeping heart disease out of your life, by identifying the common, as well as not so common, markers of heart disease. This part also focuses on solid, safe, and natural preventative strategies (without the use of drugs) that you can actively and seamlessly incorporate into your lifestyle so that the risk of heart disease developing is dramatically reduced along with your arrhythmias (if you have them). And, even if you're a healthy person without heartbeat irregularities, you will learn techniques and strategies that can keep heart disease and its devastating effects out of your life.

The book is really written for the layperson. It is not overly cluttered with many citations and footnotes and it is not intended to be a medical research paper that is largely incomprehensible by the common man. Granted, I am not a medical doctor and I am not purporting to have the experience or knowledge that a medical doctor does about what he or she does best, which is the diagnosis and treatment of disease. A medical doctor's treatment of disease is primarily undertaken with drugs (many of which unfortunately are harsh with undesirable side effects), surgery and/or invasive procedures in most cases. In fact, if you are like most normal people, taking a lifetime of drugs, undergoing expensive, risky surgery or having your bodily organs probed and infiltrated is not really something you particularly relish. But, this book is not about that. It is not about symptoms, medical diagnosis and cure (which are primarily reserved for medical doctors), other than to report what has already been written.

Rather, it is about natural strategies and protocols that guide you towards taking preventative measures to curtail, suppress or stop a health problem. This is accomplished through the use of certain safe and natural nutritional supplements and the implementation of some lifestyle changes. And, when coupled with your own normal, and actually quite powerful, biological processes, spectacular results can be achieved.

Along these lines, my research has led me to the belief that medical doctors in general have not been completely and even adequately trained in preventative techniques as well as the applications and full benefits of nutritional supplements. Their skills are directed primarily towards medical problems *after* they have occurred.

Yes, I saw many doctors to treat my heartbeat irregularity problem but all of them came up short of finding the complete solution. In every encounter with the mainstream medical community, I was confronted with either a lifetime of expensive drugs, worrisome invasive procedures or the notion of "just having to live with it." This wasn't good enough for me. Indeed, I felt that either the medical community had let me down.

For quite some time, like most Americans, I had the mistaken belief that as long as you can afford modern medicine, just go to "your doctor" and the doctor can fix the problem. Unfortunately, I had placed my expectations of the medical community at too high a level. Over time, it has become readily apparent to me that medical doctors do not cure every medical problem that they see and frequently do not meet patient expectations. As a result, patients are left disappointed and abandoned by the mainstream medical community.

I indeed became disappointed and disenchanted with the medical community. I knew that there had to be a better way and I knew that I had to be proactive in correcting my heart arrhythmias. After all, I had been proactive before with respect to a major medical problem and it worked and I felt I could do it again.

While I am not a medical doctor, I am highly educated. I have received my juris doctor and also have a specialist degree beyond my law degree (it's called a Master of Laws). I am also a co-author of three other books (both of which took complicated legal issues and made them easy to understand for the layperson). And, I was also a former trial lawyer for the U.S. Treasury Department. Trial law in large part involves taking a massive amount of difficult technical materials and information and making it comprehensible so a court of law can understand. Moreover, in my law practice, I have seen many clients die and I have usually investigated why they die and how they could have lived a healthier, more productive life. I have observed several common denominators in connection with people dying and how death may have been prevented. Indeed, I have spent the better part of the past 15 years reading books, magazines, research papers, and journals on the instant subject matter. I researched everything I could pertaining to heart arrhythmias, and as a natural corollary, heart health in general. I tested several natural strategies and found that they not only worked but they had some very positive side effects and virtually no negative side effects. I also interviewed physicians, pharmacists, scientists, researchers and nutritionists on the topic about which you are to read – notably heart arrhythmias and general heart health. Yes, I have had heart arrhythmias and I have gotten them under control!

Most medical articles and papers are difficult to read and comprehend. So, one of my objectives in writing this book was to take a specific area of your bodily process (notably your heartbeat within your cardiovascular system) and first, provide a simple explanation of the basic operation of certain aspects of your heart. Secondly, I endeavored to examine heartbeat irregularities that exist in otherwise healthy individuals. I learned that there were millions of people with this condition – a condition that can be most disconcerting. I wanted to provide some easy-to-understand, easy-to-implement, common sense ideas and suggestions in terms of addressing this problem. The breadth of this project actually grew beyond my expectations, as I was able to uncover many safe and natural preventative strategies dealing with heart health in general.

I have personally undertaken and implemented all of the suggestions discussed in this book in terms of preventing irregular heartbeats and preventing heart disease in general. My strategies and techniques have been monitored by several of my colleagues and medical doctors, including family practitioners, cardiologists and electrocardiophysiologists. I believe I am well qualified to write about my experiences and travails with respect to heartbeat irregularities and the many natural and safe ways to prevent them as well as achieving pristine cardiovascular health.

While much of the information and recommendations in this book is straightforward, intuitively correct and easily implemented, there are strategies and suggestions that may seem unfamiliar or new to you – hopefully, refreshingly new. In either event, I hope that all of the ideas should at least inspire you to proactively take steps to improve the state of your cardiovascular health from a preventative standpoint and utilize the information in a manner that best serves you, whether it involves immediate implementation or further independent investigation.

My ultimate goal in writing this book is to provide you with clearly stated strategies and guidelines that can afford you the opportunity to have all parts of your entire cardiovascular system working correctly and harmoniously in a safe and natural manner.

PART I

Heart Palpitations and Arrhythmias

Introduction to Part I

"There is no use whatever trying to help people who do not help themselves. You cannot push anyone up a ladder unless he be willing to climb himself."

—Andrew Carnegie

Before I state what the objective of the first part of this book is all about, let's talk about what it is not. This book is not directly about the diagnosis, treatment and cure of heart disease. That is a subject for a trained, licensed medical professional. There are many heart conditions that competent cardiologists are licensed to deal with every day.

The purpose of Part I of this book is to shed some light on certain heart irregularities, provide information that should have the effect of reducing the stress and panic level when the heart palpitations and arrhythmias occur, and suggest some natural preventative and relief measures, which do not involve drugs, and do not involve surgery or other invasive procedures. There are so many people like me who to their knowledge have strong healthy hearts, but for "some reason" have non-rhythmic beats occurring from time to time. And, they can be very disconcerting. If you are not knowledgeable about them, they can cause you to think you are actually having a heart attack.

I remember my first bout with atrial fibrillation in 1991, a type of irregular heartbeat that I will describe in much greater detail below. I was in Las Vegas at the airport taking the "red eye" back to Dallas. I was nibbling on some popcorn and sipping some beverage at the bar while waiting for my flight and all of a sudden, it overcame me – a wild, irregular, rapid heartbeat. I contacted the authorities at the airport and they called for an ambulance, with respect to which took an eternity, so it seemed. I was alone and had no idea what was happening. I thought I was having a heart attack. Of course, I was experiencing atrial fibrillation. The ambulance came, and to make a long story short, I spent the better part of the next 9 hours in the emergency room at a Las Vegas hospital. Eventually, the condition subsided and I was released at 9:30 AM the next morning – tired,

3

drained and worried about what happened. Certainly, this was a very scary experience and one that I am sure many of you can relate to if you have ever had atrial fibrillation.

Nearly 10 million Americans suffer from arrhythmia, or an alteration in the rhythm of the heartbeat either in the timing of the beat or the force of it. Many of these people (in excess of 2.2 million) have no apparent traces of serious heart disease. While traditional medical treatments emphasize dangerous anti-arrhythmia drugs, implantable defibrillators, and other invasive procedures, the focus here is to provide you with an extremely effective arrhythmia prevention and suppression program. You will be asked to follow some simple lifestyle modification recommendations and nutritional techniques. This program is the culmination of many long years of study and experimentation by me.

Again, this is not to act as a substitute for treatment by a licensed cardiologist or other medical specialist if you have one of the many forms of heart disease. If you have a heart condition, see your doctor. However, in many cases, several of the recommended lifestyle modifications and nutritional suggestions can be implemented right along with your doctor's advice.

Most everyone reading this book has experienced (or has had a loved one experience) the frightening situation where your/their heart sort of hiccups, flutters, or beats rapidly or irregularly. Anyone who has experienced this has undergone every possible emotion, from serious concern all the way to total panic.

If you go to your doctor, they probably will diagnose the situation, and if you have no apparent heart abnormality, they probably will conclude that it just has to be monitored. Some doctors will give you drugs, such as beta or alpha blockers, which has a tendency of slowing down and/or regulating the heart rate and blood pressure. Other doctors may prescribe stronger anti-arrhythmia medicine that can potentially eliminate the problem, but along with it come a host of potential side effects such as creating other arrhythmias. Still others might talk about catheter ablation, pacemakers, electroshock therapy, and even open heart surgery.

But, all this does not consider that in many cases you are not in a position to go to your doctor when you have a problem. Typically, an irregular heartbeat does not occur during normal business hours. It can strike at any time, and typically after normal business hours. So, you are typically faced with having to go to the emergency room at the hospital, go through the many tests, procedures, IV's and long waits in between. Each time you go you incur hundreds, and in most cases, thousands of dollars of charges. Hopefully, you have good insurance, because this can get rather expensive, not to mention your having to go through an uncomfortable, anxious, drawn out and downright irritating situation.

Is this something that you want? Obviously, it is not. You ask, is there a better way? Well, there is, and it is easy and inexpensive – and is described in detail in this book!

Chapter 1
Heart Basics 101

"Pain makes man think. Thought makes man wise. Wisdom makes life endurable."

—John Patrick

Before I begin to provide you with solutions in connection with arrhythmias, I must explain how the problems come about in the first place. In this chapter I will focus on how your heart works and how the electrical system in your heart causes both regular and irregular beats. After you learn the basics about how your heart works, I will move on to the next chapter on your heart rate.

THE HARDEST WORKER YOU WILL EVER KNOW

Picture yourself applying for a job and your prospective employer says that you can have the job, although you must work 24 hours a day, 7 days a week, non-stop with no breaks and no lunch hours. In fact, there is so much work to do, there is no time off on weekends, no vacations and no personal days or anything like that. The job is so labor intensive that you are not allowed to go anywhere else at anytime. You will stay in the same place, day after day and do the same thing over and over, and if you stop working, there are severe, virtually fatal penalties. As for compensation, what if your prospective employer said we will only pay you room and board – and the food may not even be that healthy for you.

Sound like something anyone in his or her right mind would want? Well, obviously, this is more of a nightmare than a job description. However, in reality this is the "job description" of the work of your heart – a lonely, tireless and under-appreciated job that most often is taken for granted.

Indeed, the human heart pumps approximately 100,800 times every day (about 2,000 gallons of blood each day), or about 70 times a minute in the average adult. That's over 30 million times per year and in the average lifespan of 80, it's approximately 2.4 billion beats. With each heartbeat, the bloodstream transports oxygen and nutrients to the approximately 300 trillion cells in your body in order to stay alive – 24 hours a day, 7 days a week – in an efficient manner. In fact, your entire circulatory system is so intricate that if you lay out your system of arteries and veins end to end, they would stretch over 100,000 miles! In other words, your cardiovascular system of blood flow would stretch around the earth twice, yet your blood completes an entire cycle of flow about once a minute.

Now, that is a lot of work! And, your heart doesn't ask for much. Just a little caring – moderate exercise (to keep it strong to prevent the conduction system from deteriorating) and stay away from trans and many (but not all) saturated fats and don't smoke. That sounds like "dirt cheap" wages, but most people neither have the drive nor the motivation, let alone the information to pay these "wages" and, as a consequence, they lead a life of heart disease inevitability.

THE MAKE-UP AND FUNCTION OF THE HEART MUSCLE

Your heart is a single organ muscle, but functions primarily as a double-sided pump. It is mainly designed to bring oxygen to all parts of your body. The left side of your heart pumps blood rich in oxygen to all parts of your body (initially through your aorta, which is the large blood vessel attached to your heart muscle). Your veins and capillaries carry the oxygen-depleted blood to the right side of your heart first before it can go to your lungs to pick up more oxygen.

As noted, although your heart is a single organ, it is composed of several different structures. Let's break down the role and function of each of these structures. *Coronary arteries* deliver blood to your heart muscle. *Valves* (two on each side of the heart) direct blood flow in and out of your heart and among its four chambers: two upper (atria) and two lower (ventricles).

The *right atrium* receives blood from your body. The *left atrium* receives oxygenated blood from your lungs. The *right ventricle* pumps blood to your lungs for fresh oxygen, whereas the *left ventricle* pumps oxygenated blood around your body.

The *pericardium* is the sheath or envelope on the outside that covers and protects your heart muscle. The septum is a muscle down the center of the heart. It separates the right side, where blood returns from your body on its way to your lungs to refresh its oxygen content, from the left, where the oxygen-rich blood is pumped out to the rest of your body.

However, even if you provide some caring to your heart, it still may not be as reliable as you would like. You still have that flip-flop feeling you get sometimes while lying in bed. Or, that pounding in the chest you felt when you got stressed out on a project at work or when your spouse drives you to the brink. When is irregular or rapid heart rhythm just a passing, harmless phenomenon and when is it a sign of real trouble?

HEARTBEAT VARIATION

The good news is that we all have some measure of irregularity to our heartbeats, and no one's heart rhythm is perfectly regular. In fact, my cardiologist once told me that if people grew old enough, everyone would have a heart rhythm abnormality.

Actually, variation of the heartbeat (as compared with an irregular heart beat) is really a desirable feature of heart rhythm that indicates good overall health. And, believe it or not, the most physically fit athletes, just as an example, have the greatest degree of heartbeat variation! And, if this will make you feel even better, heartbeat variation is a reflection of the parasympathetic nervous system manifesting itself, which is the subconscious control system that encourages low blood pressure and feelings of relaxation and calm. Folks who meditate or use biofeedback can ratchet up their parasympathetic tone and thereby increase their beat-to-beat variation in heart rate.

In fact, a lack of beat-to-beat variation can suggest latent dangers and the potential for heart attack and even death. I am sure you have known or have observed terribly unhealthy people, who look overweight, who eat horribly, and who even smoke and they have no claim of problem with their heartbeat. Paradoxically, if it is any consolation to you (while it should be tremendously disconcerting news for them), your occasionally irregular heartbeat is a sign of a much healthier heart than theirs!

Now, if at this point you are jumping up for joy, shouting "Gee, I am actually not that bad after all", I encourage you to now relax and read on. The information in this book is quite fascinating and should hopefully be the harbinger of a new refreshing outlook, sort of a new beginning, for you in connection with the irregular heartbeat problem of yourself or that of someone you know.

Now, as noted above, variation of your heart rhythm in and of itself is not *per se* a sign of heart disease. At some point, however, your heart's rhythm can exceed its controls and violate healthy limits of variability. This is when you have a situation going on called an "arrhythmia" or "palpitation."

As suggested, some arrhythmias are benign and simply an annoyance (easy for me to say when your heart feels as though it is jumping and even racing, but I too have "been there, done that" many times). Other arrhythmias, however, are not so harmless and can actually be life threatening. So, the question is how can you tell the difference? And, what natural, non-medicinal and non-invasive strategies can be implemented as a safe alternative to traditional medical therapies that, to be frank, can be quite scary. Later in this book I will disclose seven nutritional and strategies techniques to keep your heart in rhythm.

But, first, let's discuss some basics of your heart rate as well as the make up of your heart muscle. My intent is to provide you with a layperson's understanding of these areas, since they are vital in laying the foundation to suggesting some natural corrective measures covered later in the book.

HOW THE HEART'S ELECTRICAL CONDUCTION SYSTEM WORKS

To better understand the mechanism and characteristics of heartbeat irregularities, I will begin by describing the normal electrical activity of your heart.

As stated above, there are four chambers, two upper chambers called the left and the right atria and two lower chambers known as the right and left ventricles. Separating these upper and lower chambers there are valves that passively open and close to direct the flow of blood. The left ventricle performs the most work and is the strongest of the chambers because it ejects blood into your aorta (the main pipeline that supplies oxygenated blood to your entire body).

The electrical system of your heart consists of pathways that deliver the signals to keep your heart beating. In order for your heart to pump, it must receive some electrical stimulation that will cause the muscle to contract to generate the pumping. During a normal heartbeat, an electrical impulse originates in a particular area of your right atrium called the *sinoatrial node*. This is called the "SA node" for short. This impulse travels simultaneously to your left atrium as well as down the middle of the top part of your heart called the *interatrial septum* to the lower part of your heart called the *atrioventricular node* (AV node for short). The electrical impulse slows down briefly at this point and then continues to travel down right between your two ventricles and then breaks off and sort of surrounds each of your ventricles. (Again, to use cardiology jargon, the electrical impulse splits off into the right and left "bundle branches" located in both ventricles).

This cycle of electrical stimulation is known as normal sinus rhythm ("NSR" for short), which describes a form of natural synchronization between your atria and the ventricles of your heart, producing the normal heart sounds you hear and certainly expect to hear. In this connection, it is important to remember the SA node, because it represents the place where your normal heartbeat rhythm is initiated.

However, blocked or erratic signals interfere with normal muscle contraction, causing your heart muscle to beat too quickly or irregularly – leading to possible heart block, cardiac arrest, ventricular fibrillation, or the less dangerous premature ventricular contractions or the below-described lone atrial fibrillation.

YOUR HEART RATE: WHAT'S NORMAL AND WHAT'S ABNORMAL

The term "normal heart rate" is somewhat of an oxymoron, since heart rates range widely, depending on a number of factors – age, fitness level, mood, physical activity, and fluid intake (particularly the degree to which you consume caffeinated beverages). A heart rate that is considered normal ranges from as low as 50 beats per minute to as high as 99 beats per minute. Rates at the lower end suggest fitness (those athletes where cardiovascular exercise is predominant). On the other hand, heart rates can decline with age, as the heart's conduction system slowly degenerates, resulting in the need for pacemakers in some people. That is why you must keep your heart strong and healthy. After all, after beating 1 to 2 billion times (non-stop, with no rest), doesn't it seem logical that your heart might wear down a bit if you are not careful?

Rates at the either end (of the 50-99 beats per minute range) can suggest, but not be conclusive about, latent medical problems, such as dehydration, thyroid disorders, infections, and anxiety. In other words, higher heart rates within the "normal" range are not indicative of any particular problem, but can be a symptom of illnesses or other problems not directly involving the heart. Anecdotally, a 2000 study showed that there were two characteristics of otherwise healthy people that died suddenly from cardiac arrest: (i) resting heart rates in excess of 75 beats per minute, and (ii) a heart rate that does not easily reduce itself after exercise.[1]

Heart rates that are less than or greater than the normal range of 50-99 beats per minute are clearly abnormal and should be addressed by a doctor – ideally a cardiologist. While there is little that can be done to influence the development of a slower heart rhythm (other than taking on a more extensive aerobic exercise program), there are some things that can be done to address rapid or demonstrably irregular heart rhythms.

SYMPTOMS OF IRREGULAR HEART BEATS

As noted above, palpitations by themselves are exceptionally common and not necessarily related to your heart's rhythm. Being aware of palpitations or the flip-flop feeling in your chest, without feeling faint or losing consciousness, can suggest the presence of an arrhythmia. But, if you have felt faint, or passed out from an arrhythmia, then your condition takes on a new meaning. In this latter situation, your medical doctor will try to record and monitor your heart rhythms with such devices as "halter monitors", electrocardiograms, and ultrasound.

The bottom line here is that your heart must be able to do its job continuously without interruption or rest – that is, to pump blood throughout your body. If your heart beats too slow or too fast, or is irregular or simply out of sync, it may struggle to do its job. When your heart is unable to pump blood optimally (particularly to your lungs and brain), you can become lightheaded, breathless and even lose consciousness. In the worst case, particularly if your heart structure is significantly abnormal, some arrhythmias can be fatal.

THE IMPORTANCE OF LEARNING ABOUT THE STRUCTURE OF YOUR OWN HEART MUSCLE

When you have an episode of irregular or rapid heartbeat, the normal question to ask is, "do I have a serious problem here?" If you have damaged heart muscle or abnormal heart structure, such as that resulting from a previous heart attack or viral infection, or some congenital defect, then your rapid heart rhythm can be potentially dangerous, and even life threatening. However, the difficulty is that someone with the same type of symptoms may have a normal heart structure with a rather benign arrhythmia that represents little or no danger and one that can easily be treated. In other words, the same heart rate, and even the same rhythm, can have very different implications, depending on the underlying state of your heart. The real issue revolves around the internal structure of your heart. Simply stated, are there any defective working parts? As pointed out above, this question should be answered by a licensed physician. Usually this will be accomplished by imaging the heart with tests such as stress tests and ultrasound imaging.

What you have learned in Chapter 1 is that your heart is the quintessential tireless worker, spending its entire existence working 24 hours a day to keep you alive and healthy. The left side pumps blood enriched with oxygen from your lungs to all parts of your body. The right side receives oxygen-depleted blood from your veins and capillaries before it goes to your lungs to get more oxygen.

Your heart is a complex organ and needs electrical stimulation to continuously pump blood to where it is supposed to go in your body. Variation in heartbeat and even occasional irregularity is not unexpected in normal, healthy people. In fact, it is very common in healthy adults.

The master pacemaker in your heart is at the sinoatrial node, or SA node for short. This part of your heart makes sure that your heart beats regularly and evenly; normal being anywhere from 50–99 beats per minute.

If your beat is irregular, unaccompanied by other symptoms, such as fainting, dizziness or shortness of breath, your situation is not that bad, although definitely worthy of being checked out by a doctor, particularly if you have never had it checked out before. Similarly, if you have irregular heartbeats and have had previous heart disease, then it could mean that something serious is going on.

Chapter 2
The Most Common Irregular Heartbeats

In Chapter 2, I will identify the most common heartbeat irregularities and explain how they occur and what happens to your heart when they occur. I will also discuss the impact of these irregular beats in your body. By the time you finish reading this chapter, you should be much more knowledgeable about irregular beats that are somewhat harmless and those that should be of more serious concern to you. If you have the benign harmless type of arrhythmias, then you should gain greater peace of mind knowing that your situation is not so grave and can be treated with natural and safe techniques.

Any disturbance in the natural rhythm of the heart is called a cardiac arrhythmia or irregular heartbeat. The term "arrhythmia" refers to a disorder of your heart's beating rhythm. Arrhythmias are also often called "heart murmurs." They are actual depressions and accelerations in your heart rate that are not related to the normal changes in heart rate that occur during daily periods of rest and activity. In other words, your heart may seem to skip a beat or beat irregularly or very fast or very slowly.

An arrhythmia can range in severity from merely annoying to immediately life threatening. There are various different types of arrhythmias ranging from almost harmless to very serious. The correct diagnosis of the specific type and underlying condition in connection with the arrhythmia is extremely important.

Premature beats (also known as "contractions") are beats that occur earlier than expected and briefly interrupt your normal heart rhythm. Premature beats are the most common cause of an irregular heartbeat. Although they tend to be more common in people with heart disease, almost everyone experiences them at least occasionally. Premature beats often cause a sensation of a "skipped beat" or "flip-flop." What are really felt are not the premature beats themselves, but rather the forceful beat that follows the pause (one or two seconds) after the premature beat. During the pause, your heart has more time to fill with blood making the next beat more forceful. The pause, followed by a strong beat can actually feel like the heart skipped a beat. Premature beats are sometimes, but not always, associated with other arrhythmias. Premature beats may originate from anywhere in your heart.

If you experience an occasional premature or "skipped heartbeat" you should not be alarmed. Most people have felt their heart beat very fast, experienced a fluttering in their chest, or noticed that their heart skipped a beat. Almost everyone has also felt dizzy, faint, out of breath or had chest pains at one time or another. One of the most common arrhythmias is sinus arrhythmia, the change in heart rate that can occur normally when we take a breath. These experiences may cause anxiety, but for the majority of people, they are completely harmless. You should not panic if you experience a few flutters or your heart races occasionally. If you are a person with no significant abnormalities of the heart, normally you have a very low risk of having serious problems. If the arrhythmia, on the other hand, occurs on a recurring basis and lasts for more than one beat at a time, then there could be some grounds for alarm.

There are two types of arrhythmias. One is called *"tachycardia"*, when your heart beats too quickly, and *"bradycardia"*, when your heat beats too slowly. Most arrhythmias fall into the *tachycardia* category, with some originating in your ventricles and others in your atria. A type of arrhythmia called *"ventricular tachycardia"* is the most serious of the two and is the most common cause of sudden cardiac death.

As noted, palpitations generally are often not serious, although quite disconcerting. However, it depends on whether or not the sensations represent an abnormal heart rhythm (arrhythmia). You are more likely to have an abnormal heart rhythm if you have: (i) known heart disease at the time the palpitations begin, (ii) significant risk factors for heart disease, (iii) an abnormal heart valve, and (iv) an electrolyte abnormality, such as low potassium.

Some of the most common heart irregularities are called premature atrial contractions and premature ventricular contractions (PACs and PVCs, respectively) and atrial fibrillation (AFIB). In many situations they occur independently of each other. In other cases, PACs and PVCs can lead right into AFIB. It is estimated that over 2 million people in the U.S. (and millions more around the world) suffer from these arrhythmias. Some are related to serious heart conditions. However, in very many cases, these conditions can be relatively harmless.

For the purposes of ease of reference we will refer to both PACs and PVCs as PCs. The two situations that are fairly benign is where the PCs are not consecutive, one right after another. AFIB cases that are not that serious fall into the arena called "lone AFIB", which will be discussed in greater detail below, where the condition is not the result of other heart disease, but is brought on by stress, genetic make-up or other consumables which tend to trigger the arrhythmias. Occasional PCs would definitely be classified as a palpitation, whereas AFIB would ordinarily be classified as an arrhythmia. Because lone AFIB may not necessarily be part of any other heart ailment, it is difficult for it to be categorized in the class of demonstrably more serious heart arrhythmias. Whatever the categorization, sufferers worldwide know what it is like to endure bouts of PCs and lone AFIB.

While the focus of the first part of this book is to point out some of the more natural non-medical approaches to dealing with rather benign palpitations and arrhythmias, if you are having heartbeat irregularities that are accompanied by shortness of breath, chest pain, unusual sweating, dizziness, or lightheadedness, or you have fainted, call the doctor or go the emergency room. This is a sign of more serious problems. Similarly, if the PCs are very frequent (such as more than 6 per minute or in runs of 3 or more) see a medical doctor, usually a cardiologist.

PREMATURE VENTRICULAR CONTRACTIONS (PVCs)

There are other cells throughout your heart that can also generate electrical impulses. These cells can take over for your main pacemaker if they are strong enough. Some of them are located in, and come from, an irritable area in your heart's lower pumping chambers (the ventricles). If these cells fire at the wrong time, the electrical impulse they generate will cause your ventricles to contract early, resulting in a premature ventricular contraction, or PVC. PVCs are also known as *"ventricular extrasystoles,"* which means "extra" heartbeats.

In other words, the normal pace-making activity of your sinus (SA) node suppresses electric impulse production by your other cells. But if the electrical signal from your sinus (SA) node to some other part of your the heart muscle is blocked, or if your heart is over stimulated, many of these cells may express their inherent impulse-production ability, resulting in irregular beats. In other words, impulses are fired from one or more locations in addition to the normal pacemaker, the sinus node.

They may be caused by a number of factors, although the cause of PVCs in any one person is considered by the traditional medical community to be unknown.

PREMATURE ATRIAL CONTRACTIONS (PACS)

As the name suggests, premature atrial contractions (PACs) are contractions in the atria of the heart that occur too early in the rhythm sequence. They are also called *"atrial ectopic beats"*, or *"atrial extrasystoles."* Such extra beats, much like their cousin in originating in the ventricles, often occur in normal, healthy hearts and are also usually harmless. They can, however, cause palpitations, as well as trigger rapid heart rate. Many of these episodes are not serious.

Most persons who have PACs never notice them. Because PACs occur out of the normal rhythm, this condition is considered to be an arrhythmia.

PAC's originate within your atria, but outside the SA node. Typically, a PAC occurs before your next expected sinus rhythm electrical impulse. It may be conducted normally through your AV node and ventricles; or, it can be partially or completely blocked. The cause of a PAC is not fully known by the mainstream medical community. An increased rate of PACs has been observed prior to the onset of atrial fibrillation and has been associated with lung and thyroid diseases.

COMMON DENOMINATORS OF PREMATURE ATRIAL AND VENTRICULAR CONTRACTIONS

You can have PCs even if you have a healthy, normal heart. The vast majority of PCs have no symptoms, possibly with the exception of the physical feeling of a "skipped beat." PCs can increase in frequency as you get older, whether or not you have organic heart disease. In the presence of known or unknown underlying heart disease, these arrhythmias may be a harbinger for the future occurrence of an underlying cardiovascular disease such as coronary artery disease, cardiomyopathy (diseased muscle tissue), or other heart problems or incapacitating arrhythmias (other than PCs). However, if you don't have such organic heart disease, PCs have not been shown to predict the presence, or future occurrence of, clinically significant arrhythmia for you. PCs are, therefore, often considered to be harmless.

That's the good news. However, the bad news is that you still feel them and they are most disconcerting and downright scary. PCs interrupt the normal heart rhythm and cause an irregular beat. This is often felt as a "missed beat" or a "flip-flop" in your chest. But, as noted, when they occur very often or repetitively, they can lead to more serious rhythm disturbances.

If PCs are becoming troublesome, or they cannot be felt at all, continuous electrocardiographic monitoring may be necessary, especially during exercise. It may reveal more frequent and complex PCs as compared with a single routine electrocardiogram (EKG). This involves wearing a heart monitor for a period of time from several days to a few weeks while performing normal work or home activities. If episodes occur, the monitor records what has happened and can electronically transmit the information to be interpreted.

ATRIAL FIBRILLATION (AFIB)

Atrial fibrillation, which will be discussed in more detail in the next chapter, is a disorder found in about 2.2 million Americans. The likelihood of developing atrial fibrillation increases with age and affects men slightly more often than women. AFIB plagues around 10% of people age 80 and over, and is a frequent cause of hospitalization. Until just a few years ago health care providers thought AFIB to be a "nuisance" arrhythmia with few consequences. However, recent medical research has uncovered some devastating complications including stroke, congestive heart failure and cardiomyopathy that are directly related to AFIB.

Briefly, this is what happens when you have AFIB. Your atria (your heart's two small upper chambers) quiver instead of beating effectively. Blood isn't pumped completely out of them, so it may pool and clot. If a blood clot in your atria leaves the heart and becomes lodged in an artery in your brain, a stroke results. About 15 percent of strokes occur in people with AFIB.

Like PCs, research has yet to uncover the definitive cause of AFIB.

OTHER TYPES OF ARRHYTHMIAS

There are dozens of arrhythmias other than PCs and AFIB. Since I am reviewing the basics of arrhythmias, it is always helpful to spend a little time briefly understanding these other types of arrhythmias, notably those:

Originating in your Atria

Sinus arrhythmia. This involves cyclic changes in your heart rate during breathing. This ailment is common in children and often found in adults.

Sinus tachycardia. Your SA node sends out electrical signals faster than usual, speeding up your heart rate.

Sick sinus syndrome. Your SA node does not fire its signals properly, so that your heart rate slows down. Sometimes the rate changes back and forth between a slow and fast rate.

Paroxysmal atrial tachycardia (PAT). In *paroxysmal tachycardia*, repeated periods of very fast heartbeats begin and end suddenly.

Atrial flutter. Rapidly fired signals cause the muscles in your atria to contract quickly, leading to a very fast, steady heartbeat.

Wolff-Parkinson-White syndrome. Abnormal pathways between your atria and ventricles cause the electrical signal to arrive at your ventricles too soon and to be transmitted back into your atria. Very fast heart rates may develop as the electrical signal ricochets between your atria and ventricles.

Supraventricular tachycardia (SVT). *Supraventricular tachycardia* (SVT) is a general term describing any rapid heart rate originating above your ventricles, or lower chambers of your heart. SVT is an arrhythmia, or abnormal heart rhythm. Specific types of SVT actually include atrial fibrillation, AV nodal re-entrant tachycardia, and Wolff-Parkinson-White syndrome. SVT generally begins and ends quickly. Many people experience short periods of SVT and have no symptoms. However, SVT becomes a problem when it occurs frequently or lasts for long periods of time and produces symptoms.

Originating in your Ventricles

Ventricular tachycardia. Your heart beats fast due to electrical signals arising from your ventricles (rather than from your atria).

Ventricular fibrillation. Electrical signals in your ventricles are fired in a very fast and uncontrolled manner, causing your heart to quiver rather than beat and pump blood.

THE PROS AND CONS OF TRADITIONAL ANTI-ARRHYTHMIC DRUGS

The primary treatment by mainstream physicians for arrhythmias are expensive prescription drugs (particularly if you don't have adequate health insurance). For quite some time, mishaps and unexpected side effects have been associated with anti-arrhythmic prescription medications. The drug *encainide* is supposed to produce helpful effects by slowing nerve impulses in the heart and making the heart tissue less sensitive. *Encainide* was widely prescribed in the 1980's but withdrawn from the market when reports of serious adverse effects began to accumulate.

While this drug was extremely effective in suppressing arrhythmias, the most dangerous heart arrhythmias of all (which are ventricular tachycardia and fibrillation, and one known as "Torsade de Pointes") actually increased with treatment. In other words, encainide caused new heart rhythm problems when used. This example and other similar situations clearly evidence that simply suppressing irregular heartbeats may not result in better ultimate outcomes.

Moreover, it is widely recognized, by physicians and non-physicians alike, that many anti-arrhythmia medications have the risk of serious side effects. The drug *procainamide* (under the brand name *"Pronestyl"*), for example, can cause lupus-like syndrome and a whole slew of other side effects, not the least of which is an increased risk of death! Now, doesn't that make you "all warm and fuzzy."

Another drug, called *amiodarone,* has been clearly related to thyroid disorders, liver dysfunction, and incapacitating and sometimes fatal lung disease, including all of the symptoms of same, such as shortness of breath (dyspnea), cough, fever, and chest pain along with inflammation of the lung tissue (plueritis).

With a drug called *Tambocor*™, known as a Class I anti-arrhythmic drug (also known as generic under the name *flecainide*), the matter is quite simple and straightforward. The side effect here is that you have an increased risk that you will die from the use of the drug. And, under those circumstances, you can unequivocally say that your irregular heartbeat will go away – permanently! Don't run too fast to your local pharmacy to get this gem!

All sarcasm aside, there have been some very large studies on Tambocor™ and there have been reports of some very bad side effects, including the creation of additional, different arrhythmias than those diagnosed prior to taking the drug, notably increased PCs. There does seem to be some medical support (as reported in the New England Journal of Medicine) for taking this drug only when there is an attack of lone AFIB, rather than on an everyday basis (see your doctor for the correct dose). And, notice I said lone AFIB. This strategy is usually done in cases where you have an otherwise healthy heart. This is because the medical evidence seems to support the medical complications falling in the class of cases where there were some significant heart abnormalities to begin with.

Other than that, because of their risks, these drugs are reserved for the most dangerous heart arrhythmias. The imperfections and pitfalls of rhythm correcting medications have led many cardiologists to favor other techniques, such as implanted defibrillators that deliver an internal shock to the patient to terminate life-threatening arrhythmias.

There is one question that remains. If you take these drugs, or any of the anti-arrhythmia medicines for that matter, for a short time and then stop the drug, will you nevertheless, retain the new arrhythmias you acquired when you took the drug, if you in fact "inherited" new arrhythmias in the first place? Your doctor will probably tell you that you will only have this risk when you take the medicine. This fact still remains to be verified.

To summarize Chapter 2, there are many types of heart arrhythmias, ranging from harmless to life threatening. When these arrhythmias are happening, the electrical impulses that naturally occur in other parts of your heart overwhelm your main pacemaker (the SA node) and interfere with your normal sinus rhythm. While you should have some knowledge of most arrhythmias, my focus in this book is mainly benign premature ventricular contractions, premature atrial contractions and atrial fibrillation. Even though these benign arrhythmias are relatively harmless and not life-threatening, they can be extremely trouble-some from a mental, emotional and physiological standpoint. Moreover, if you are having heartbeat irregularities that are accompanied by shortness of breath, chest pain, unusual sweating, dizziness, or lightheadedness, or you have fainted, this is a sign of more serious problems and you should seek medical attention. But, if you suffer from irregular heartbeats unaccompanied by other symptoms, it is important for you to be able to control them, prevent them from happening and reduce their impact on your life. Conventional medicine typically prescribes drugs, which are quite expensive and far from the perfect solution.

As noted, PCs are fairly harmless, and usually AFIB is harmless as well, although in some situations it can develop into something more serious if certain precautions are not taken. Chapter 3 discusses AFIB in more detail and describes what the traditional medical community is doing about this condition.

Chapter 3
Atrial Fibrillation in Operation

"Fear is the main source of superstition, and one of the main sources of cruelty. To conquer fear is the beginning of wisdom."

—Bertrand Russell

In Chapter 3, you will learn how AFIB interrupts your normal sinus rhythm. And, did you know that there are several types of AFIB? You will learn which are the most important for you to be concerned about. And, conventional medicine has a variety of techniques to treat symptoms of AFIB. So, what are the objectives of such techniques? And, are they effective and long lasting? Also, are the risks and complications worth it? I think you'll be surprised at what the mainstream medical community has to offer.

HOW AFIB INTERRUPTS NORMAL SINUS HEART RHYTHM

In general, AFIB represents the loss of synchrony or coordination between the atria and the ventricles. Typically, AFIB is characterized as a storm of electrical energy that travels in waves across both atria, causing these upper chambers to quiver or to fibrillate at 300 to 600 times per minute. It is like the feeling you get when you are flying on an airplane through intense turbulent airspace.

As noted below, in Chapter 4, AFIB can be brought on by a host of different circumstances, including inherent heart disease, certain types of exercise or sensitivities to certain foods, beverages or drugs. When AFIB starts, the objective is to get it under control as soon as possible. Ideally, this should occur within as little as a few short minutes to up to no more than nine hours. The main purpose of controlling AFIB is to prevent blood clots resulting in heart attack or stroke.

For many years, AFIB was believed to be a completely chaotic event with unorganized electrical impulses bouncing around the atria randomly. However, modern research and computerized mapping techniques have provided greater insight into the mechanism of AFIB. Typically, there are at least six different locations in the left and right atria where relatively large circular waves of electrical currents can occur, creating a pattern of continuous electrical activity that is characteristic of complex AFIB. This important discovery paved the way for the development of a surgical technique that is designed to extinguish atrial fibrillation, notably the *Maze procedure* described in the latter part of this chapter.

AFIB can also occur as a secondary event. As an example, I discussed a trigger mechanism in the previous chapter called a premature atrial contraction (PAC), which has been associated with the initiation of AFIB in some patients.

SPECIFIC TYPES OF ATRIAL FIBRILLATION

There are many types of AFIB. The type of AFIB I am primarily focusing on in this book is one that does not appear to be associated with any identifiable cause or abnormalities of your heart. In other words, you are otherwise considered to be healthy. Medical professionals would call this "lone atrial fibrillation" or "lone AFIB." In other words, the condition is AFIB all to itself. As noted in more detail below, lone AFIB could be caused by an allergic reaction to food, drink, drugs, stress, or the result of a congenital defect.

✓AFIB, which occurs intermittently, is called *paroxysmal AFIB* and varies in frequency and duration from a few seconds to more protracted episodes lasting several hours or even days. *Lone* or *paroxysmal AFIB* tend to be seen more often in younger people aged 30-50 years. *Persistent AFIB* on the other hand, becomes a primary heart rhythm and is usually unresponsive to medical therapy or other non-pharmacologic interventions such as electrical cardioversion. This form of AFIB is typically seen in the elderly.

Early genetic research on *familial AFIB*, a relatively uncommon type of AFIB often affecting younger people (less than 20 years of age) has identified a specific chromosomal defect that is responsible for this form of arrhythmia.

Neurogenic AFIB indicates an imbalance in the nervous system regulation of your heart. One type of *neurogenic AFIB*, called *vagal AFIB*, occurs in conjunction with an enhanced, extraordinary response from a particular nerve in your heart, called the *vagus* nerve. Stimulation of your *vagus* nerve causes your heart rate to slow down and the refractory period (rest period) of the atria to shorten. Typically, *vagal AFIB* occurs more frequently when you rest or after one of your meals. If you are between the ages of 30 and 50 years of age, you fall into the group where this condition is most often observed. Sometimes this type of AFIB may be preceded by a period of a progressively slow heart rate. This is why certain medications, such as beta blockers or an anti-arrhythmic drug called *digitalis* may actually worsen the AFIB.

Adrenergic AFIB is another type of *neurogenic AFIB* that occurs typically during the day and is the result of excessive adrenaline that comes from stimulation of the sympathetic portion ("fight or flight" response) of your nervous system. When you become stressed, whether physically, mentally, or emotionally, this will affect your heart by increasing the rate and force of contraction. Unlike the case of vagal AFIB, the traditional medical community finds that beta blockers may be quite helpful in controlling this form of atrial fibrillation.

THE IMPACT OF AFIB ON YOUR LIFE

A broad range of physical symptoms may be associated with AFIB. You may have absolutely no awareness of being in atrial fibrillation, or you may know precisely the moment when your heart rhythm destabilizes from normal sinus rhythm to AFIB. The irregular, often rapid pulsations of your heart in AFIB can be described as an uncomfortable flopping sensation inside of your chest with a sudden and keen awareness of every one of your heartbeats. In cases where you could have some further serious problem (not typically associated with lone AFIB) this may be accompanied by shortness of breath, profuse sweating, chest pain, dizziness, passing out, exercise intolerance and extreme fatigue.

You also may feel anxiety and impending doom, especially when your AFIB is first discovered. If you are like some people, your pattern of atrial fibrillation may progress from a paroxysmal and infrequent event to become a chronic condition. Often, there may be a worsening or progression of your symptoms such that you may feel incapable of carrying out your normal daily activities.

For those who have not experienced AFIB, you will have difficulty understanding the impact that it can have on your daily life. Battling the physical and emotional effects of AFIB is debilitating and can lead to depression, yet no one knows that the battle exists because there are few outward physical symptoms. Employers, family members and yes, even treating physicians may be unaware of the decrease in functional capacity that AFIB causes. As a result, you often get the impression that others think you are "exaggerating" your symptoms.

Because AFIB is so unpredictable, you may be often reluctant to travel and may even avoid committing to social engagements. Frequent trips to the hospital for repeated episodes of AFIB can completely disrupt your life, causing significant emotional and physical distress to yourself and your family alike. It is for these reasons that this book is being written – to allow present sufferers of lone AFIB and even some sufferers of other forms of AFIB (who have had a history of the condition) and interested potential sufferers (and anyone who reads this book is a potential sufferer eventually) to be able to undertake steps now to prevent or reduce the chances of its occurrence and, when it does occur, to minimize its consequences and shorten its duration.

If it will make you feel any better, it is really just a matter of time before you develop this rather potentially problematical condition (if you already don't have AFIB). In fact, cardiologists aptly state that if everyone lived long enough, everyone would develop AFIB. Therefore, it would be wise to pay close attention to the preventative techniques set forth in Chapter 5 below.

HOW IS AFIB TREATED BY THE TRADITIONAL MEDICAL COMMUNITY

In general, if you don't have any independent symptoms other than the irregular heartbeat bothering you, and have no associated cardiac disease (lone AFIB), no therapy is normally indicated. If the irregular heartbeat is frequent or symptomatic, medication and other treatment is normally recommended. Such treatment options include prescription medications, electrical cardioversion, ablations, pacemakers, and surgery. Research on atrial defibrillators is ongoing for certain types of AFIB. The choice of therapy is quite individualized, after consulting with your doctor, and is usually based on the degree of disability and symptoms associated with the AFIB.

Essentially, there are three major goals of conventional medical treatment of AFIB: (i) the restoration of normal sinus rhythm, (ii) the control of the ventricular rate during AFIB, and (iii) the prevention of blood clot formation.

Treatment with Drugs

Restoring Normal Sinus Rhythm

Sinus rhythm is often restored with medications that impede the conduction of electrical impulses and decrease the excitability and the apparent independent action of cardiac cells that overpower the main pacemaker of your heart. These medications are intended to also prolong the rest period (called "*refractory period*") of cardiac tissue. Several medications may be used to terminate atrial fibrillation including *procainimide (Pronestyl), quinidine, disopyramide (Norpace), amiodarone (Cordarone), and dofetilide (Tikosyn)*. The effectiveness of these drugs and one's tolerance of drug therapy is quite individualized. Medications may often be changed in order to achieve the desired outcome of reducing the episodes of AFIB. Unfortunately, some of these drugs can have pro-arrhythmic effects, causing the heart to become even more irritable and setting the stage for new arrhythmias to occur!

Control of Ventricular Rate

To effectively reduce the symptoms associated with AFIB, the ventricular rate must be controlled. The irregular, flopping sensation in your chest that is so uncomfortable and worrisome to you, if you are an AFIB sufferer, is *not* from the irregular atrial beat, but rather is from the irregular ventricular beat in response to the AFIB. In fact, you are not capable of feeling your atria beating, only the ventricles. So, the faster your ventricles contract, the more symptoms you experience. The goal of medications such as beta blockers, calcium channel blockers, and digoxin is to slow down your heart rate by decreasing the excitability of your cardiac cells and by slowing the conduction of the electrical impulses through your AV node.

The problem with this strategy, however, is that many people with lone AFIB are generally quite healthy, with good heart rates, even very low "athletic" heart rates in the 50-59 beats per minute (resting) range. When these beta-blockers and calcium channel blockers are administered, the heart rate can proceed into the 40s, which can be, in and of itself, disconcerting. Also, this can be accompanied by lethargy and tiredness. Dizziness and even sleep disturbances can occur.

Remember, the AV node that is located between your atria and your ventricles has a protective "gatekeeper" mechanism that only allows so many impulses to travel through to your ventricles. The goal of medical therapy is to simply use the AV node's gatekeeper properties to reduce your heart's ventricular rate to 65-90 beats per minute during an episode of AFIB. The idea here is that even though your heartbeat is irregular, it is better to be irregular at 65-90 beats per minute than to be irregular at 120-150 beats per minute. This rate control in turn, decreases the workload of your heart and the symptoms of discomfort associated with a fast irregular heartbeat. Some of the medications used to produce this effect include *sotalol (Betapace), propafenone (Rythmol), propranolol (Inderal), diltiazem (Cardizem), verapamil (Calan), and digoxin (Lanoxin).*

Control of the rate at which your ventricles contract in AFIB is also important in that a prolonged rapid heart rate can actually cause a permanent physiological change to take place in your cardiac cells. These cells can cause the modification of how your heart contracts and can cause new and more serious heart conditions. This can be difficult to regulate, in that your heart rate is controlled with medication while at rest, but quickly exceeds the desired range as soon as you become moderately active. Conversely, as noted above, medication that may be prescribed to control your heart rate during activity can cause your heart to slow excessively when you are at rest. An ongoing challenge for the mainstream medical community is to fine-tune a patient's prescription drug medication regimen in order to achieve a balance between reducing the discomfort and minimizing adverse physiologic changes that can occur with poorly-controlled ventricular rates when the patient is in AFIB. This is an art form that cardiologists continue to wrestle with and is clearly an imperfect science.

Prevention of Blood Clot Formation

During AFIB, your atria lose their organized pumping action and fibrillate (quiver) in response to the continuous electrical stimulation. In normal sinus rhythm, your atria contract, the valves open and blood fills your ventricles (the lower chambers). Your ventricles then contract to complete the organized cycle of contraction that occurs with each heartbeat. Since your atria do not contract during AFIB, your blood is not able to empty efficiently from your atria into your ventricles with each heartbeat. Blood can then pool and become stagnant in your atria, creating a site for blood clot formation. Since the left side of your heart pumps the oxygenated blood to all parts of your body, clot formation in the left atrium can become a primary source of stroke for you if you are in AFIB.

One type of stroke occurs when a blood clot travels to your brain and lodges in a vessel causing the normal blood flow to stop and your brain tissue to die from lack of oxygen (in medical parlance, it's called *thromboembolic cerebral vascular accident, or CVA*). This serious complication of AFIB occurs approximately six times more often in the elderly (usually 65 and above). Thus, AFIB can pose a substantial and potentially devastating risk particularly for this age group.

Research has demonstrated that anticoagulation with a drug called "warfarin" (Coumadin) is effective in reducing the risk of blood clot formation and stroke, but it does not totally eliminate the risk. An anticoagulant or blood thinner such as Coumadin interferes with your body's normal clotting mechanism. The dosage of Coumadin has to be highly individualized and must be carefully monitored with blood tests to ensure safety.

Aspirin is an anti-platelet drug that is also used for stroke prevention. Aspirin, in low doses, decreases the stickiness of your circulating *platelets* (which are small blood cells that initiate the normal clotting process), so they will not adhere to one another and thus reduces the likelihood of forming blood clots. Aspirin is much safer than Coumadin because it is less likely to cause abnormal bleeding, including even strokes from bleeding due to the Coumadin itself. However, current research, as it pertains to traditional medicine, indicates that aspirin is *not* as effective in preventing blood clots (and therefore, strokes) as Coumadin. Using aspirin for heart disease has been controversial for years. Sure, aspirin can help in connection with blood thinning. But, the catch is that if you take aspirin there is some serious question whether your system is utilizing it properly, so you may be getting little or no protection from it. According to a study in *Circulation: Journal of the American Heart Association*, people who are aspirin-resistant have a higher risk of dying from heart disease than people who are not aspirin resistant. Additional studies show that people who are diagnosed with heart failure and follow a treatment regimen that includes blood thinners such as aspirin or Coumadin could actually be putting their health into more danger!

While millions of people take these medications every day, many suffer from a long list of side effects that include gastrointestinal bleeding and ruptured blood vessels. One only needs to look at the facts for proof – since the introduction of these medicines, there has been no decrease in the number of heart attacks and strokes in the United States!

Treatment without Drugs

Electrical Cardioversion

Electrical cardioversion, otherwise known as electro-shock therapy, is used to stop the current occurrence of AFIB, but in and of itself has no long-term effect on its recurrence. You would generally be admitted as an outpatient to the hospital (if you were not already admitted), placed on a heart monitor, an intravenous form of anesthetic is given and patches are placed on the chest.

Once you are completely anesthetized, a small electrical charge over your heart is delivered. This electrical charge causes a momentary electrical discharge of all of your cardiac cells and allows your primary pacemaker to take control of the rhythm, thus stopping your AFIB and resetting your heart. Sometimes this is done in conjunction with anti-arrhythmic medications to reduce the likelihood of recurrence of the AFIB.

Ablations for Specific Arrhythmias

Another type of treatment is called an ablation. Webster un-inspiringly defines an ablation as a "surgical excision or amputation of a body part or tissue." Ablation procedures are used to halt arrhythmias by introducing catheters into your heart (which are started through a vein in the lower torso of your body) and directing energy at specific areas of heart tissue found to be the source of the irregular rhythms. An electrophysiology (EP) study is performed to discover the location and the characteristics of the arrhythmia. Once the specific location is mapped out, then special catheters are precisely placed, radio frequency (RF) energy is passed down the catheter to the heart tissue and the tissue is destroyed. The tissue is no longer able to initiate or to conduct any type of electrical impulse. In other words, part of your heart muscle is intentionally destroyed. If you have the courage and the money to do this, ask your doctor if you have one of the conditions that are amenable to ablation therapy.

Other Types of Ablation for the Treatment of AFIB

There are other types of ablation. One involves a catheter ablation of your AV node to modify your ventricular response to AFIB. This therapy is usually employed if you are a person with a rapid heart rate that is not well controlled with medications and with symptoms related to the uncontrolled heart rate. The procedure destroys certain of the tissue at your AV node and this stops the conduction of all electrical impulses from the atria to the ventricles. In other words, this procedure disconnects the problematical electrical pathways that are near the bottom of the heart.

So, now that you have turned off certain of your tissue at, around and/or near your heart's "circuit breaker" so to speak (which does not sound too good in and of itself), what happens next? Well, ablation of your AV node requires the placement of a permanent pacemaker at the time of the procedure. The pacemaker then provides you with a steady and regular heartbeat that often diminishes the symptoms associated with your AFIB (when it works, of course), even though the atria continue to fibrillate. It is commonly recognized amongst physicians that this procedure does *not* cure the AFIB nor does it diminish the risk of stroke and therefore, anticoagulation medicine would typically be continued after the procedure. However, you may be able to reduce or discontinue medications such as beta blockers or anti-arrhythmia drugs following an AV nodal ablation because the ventricular rate is now controlled by the pacemaker. This sounds interesting but at the same time quite scary, and it doesn't seem that anyone will be "breaking down the door" to get this procedure implemented.

Pacemakers

The thought of a pacemaker for a person that perceives himself as healthy is largely viewed as being repulsive. And, as noted below, this technique is essentially reserved for people with more serious heart problems and the elderly.

Recognizably, the types of pacemakers currently in use are much more sophisticated and better capable of responding to the changing needs of your body than those that were used 15-20 years ago. The first pacemaker inserted nearly forty years ago was limited to pacing only one chamber at a fixed rate. Today's pacemakers consist of two major parts: a generator that houses a battery and electronic sensors, and the leads that connect into your heart. The generator provides a small electrical current that stimulates your heart to pump via the leads. (Remember your heart requires an electrical impulse to cause it to pump, or contract.)

The rather sophisticated built-in sensors provide continuous feedback and information from your heart, instructing the pacemaker to compensate according to your body's requirements. This allows for the pacemaker to meet your specific needs.

Pacemakers are inserted for a variety of heart conditions. (for your information examples of these conditions are called *sick sinus syndrome, supraventricular tachycardia, heart block* and *ventricular tachycardia*). The good news is that AFIB is usually not an indication for a pacemaker (whew)!

Atrial Defibrillators

Atrial defibrillators utilize specialized technology to accurately recognize AFIB and electrically convert the arrhythmia by delivering a small electrical shock via leads placed in your heart. The device is also equipped with an additional lead that provides backup pacing of your ventricle if needed. Atrial defibrillators are about the size of a conventional pacemaker and consist of a small battery pack, a generator, and three leads. The device is inserted under x-ray guidance in the cardiac catheterization laboratory by interventional cardiologists. The long term outlook for the on going use of atrial defibrillators is hard to predict.

Beyond Prescription Drugs and Traditional Procedures

The Maze Procedure

The Maze procedure is a surgical technique that cures AFIB by interrupting the circular electrical patterns or wavelets that are responsible for this arrhythmia. Yes, you read it – open-heart surgery. Your doctor will be more diplomatic by calling this a "surgical intervention."

Anyway, strategically placed incisions are made in your heart in a particular manner in both atria (very carefully, of course). This stops the formation and the conduction of irregular electrical impulses and channels the normal electrical impulse in one direction from the top of your heart to the bottom. Scar tissue generated by the incisions permanently blocks the abnormal paths of the electrical impulses that cause AFIB, thus eliminating your arrhythmia. The major advantage of this particular surgical technique over other less-invasive forms of therapy is that it corrects all three problems associated with AFIB, notably the Maze procedure: (i) ablates the arrhythmia, (ii) restores harmony between the atria and the ventricles, and (iii) preserves organized atrial contraction.

On the Horizon in the Medical Community

Technological advances and further research have recently resulted in the development of a less-invasive surgical approach for atrial fibrillation. Several research centers are currently developing specialized catheters to attempt a less invasive maze-type of procedure with ablation catheters instead of an open-heart surgical approach. There have been some early trials with this type of Maze procedure, but the results were not the best and its development continues.

A Final Thought on the Treatment of AFIB

The above discussion was really intended to describe alternative treatments for serious AFIB cases, typically accompanied by other heart disease. In a traditional sense, there is really nothing you can do for benign or lone AFIB. You can possibly take some drugs, such as beta-blockers or calcium channel blockers, but they have side effects. So, that doesn't leave much, with the exception of some natural non-medicinal suggestions on prevention and how to control AFIB and PCs, which are described in detail in Chapter 5, "The Seven Natural & Safe Ways to Protect Against Irregular Heart Beat."

So, what have we learned in Chapter 3? Typically, AFIB is characterized as a storm of electrical energy that travels in waves across both of your atria, causing these upper chambers to significantly quiver or to fibrillate. AFIB can be brought on by a host of different circumstances, including inherent heart disease or sensitivities to certain food, drink or drugs. There are many types of AFIB. The type of AFIB we are primarily focusing on in this book is one that does not appear to be associated with any identifiable cause or abnormalities of the heart. Medical professionals would call this "lone atrial fibrillation" or "lone AFIB."

AFIB can be extremely disconcerting, even if there are no accompanying symptoms such as shortness of breath, chest pain, dizziness, etc. Anxiety, panic and impending doom are all common reactions. While there are no outward symptoms, the physical and emotional effects can be quite incapacitating.

There are three major goals of conventional medical treatment with respect to the treatment of AFIB, notably the restoration of normal sinus rhythm, the control of the ventricular rate during AFIB, and the prevention of blood clot formation. This is usually handled by administering prescription drugs (nearly all of which are has worrisome negative side effects). However, many of these drugs are difficult to administer in terms of achieving the correct dosage. This is because you may be taking other drugs or agents, which interact unpredictably with the anti-arrhythmia drugs. AFIB can be also treated with electro-shock therapy, ablations (an invasive procedure where small parts of your heart is deadened to prevent unwanted electrical currents), pacemakers and atrial defibrillators, and open-heart surgery. All of these treatments are simply uninspiring and undesirable.

Thus, the best answer is to prevent them from happening in the first place. The first place to start is an analysis of causation, and this is discussed in the next chapter.

Chapter 4
What Can Cause Premature Heart Contractions, AFIB and Other Arrhythmias

"Men must try and try again. They must suffer the consequences of their own mistakes and learn by their own failures and their own successes."

—Lawson Purdy

There are many possible causes of irregular heartbeats. Can they be caused by foods, drinks, or even prescription drugs themselves? Do irregular beats happen in the same way for everyone; or, does the issue of causation become a very individualized evaluation for each person who has experienced benign arrhythmias? And, lastly, how long does it take for an irregular heartbeat symptom to manifest itself that is caused by an identifiable source? In this chapter we will discuss the most common likely causes of irregular heartbeats.

VARIOUS CAUSES

Any condition that affects the structure of your heart and your heart's electrical balance can cause a cardiac arrhythmia. If you have coronary heart disease, congenital heart defects, heart muscle disease, heart valve disorders you can easily have an arrhythmia problem. But, if your heart is otherwise structurally sound, the irregular beats can be caused by abnormalities in your body chemistry, high blood pressure or even thyroid disease. In addition, if you have a dysfunctional autonomic nervous system (meaning a poorly performing involuntary bodily function, such as the beat of your heart, or the functioning of your brain) or you

33

have lung disorders, arrhythmias can result. Arrhythmias can also be caused by external factors, like electrical shock and severe chest injury. When certain chemicals or hormones, such as caffeine, nicotine, alcohol, cocaine (and other drugs), inhaled aerosol stimulants and adrenaline, rush into your bloodstream, arrhythmias can happen.

The less life threatening heartbeat irregularities such as PVCs, PACs and lone AFIB, in addition to the above, can be caused by exercise, anxiety, stress, fear, fever, lack of quality sleep (including sleep apnea, where you actually stop breathing for as little as 10 seconds to as much as one minute during your sleep), diet pills, cough, cold medicine, anemia, hyperventilation, low levels of oxygen in your blood, and medications such as thyroid pills, asthma drugs, beta blockers for high blood pressure or heart disease, or anti-arrhythmics (medications to treat an irregular heart rhythm can sometimes cause a different irregular rhythm).

But, there can be other causes, such as allergies to certain foods (for example, dairy products, eggs, sugar, tomatoes, chocolate, alcoholic beverages and even corn, soy or garlic). Any food or other product you consume, or stressful activity you undertake, that has the effect of increasing your levels of adrenaline could be the culprit as well, since rushes of adrenaline produced by your adrenal glands is often the triggering mechanism for arrhythmias, particularly when combined with one or more of the consumables noted above. For example, you might eat a piece of sugary, rich chocolate cake right before bed. While that highly glycemic, high carb snack might be so soothing to the taste, and may even cause you to get to sleep, rushes of adrenaline two to three hours after you fall asleep could cause you to awake abruptly and actually cause you PCs or even cause your heart to go into AFIB.

And, notice I referred to soy. I will discuss this substance in greater detail in subsequent chapters, but suffice it to say at this point that soybean oil (which as you may know is contained in just about everything these days) contains high concentrations of omega-6 fatty acids.[2] These types of fatty acids actually have shown to cause palpitations.

However, each case must rest on its own facts, and many people are sensitive to different things. You need to be proactive and continually test yourself to determine which food or drink you may be consuming that triggers your particular heartbeat irregularity. Experiment by introducing and then eliminating each one that you suspect, including the suspects identified above. For example, I am sensitive to caffeine, corn, tomatoes, garlic, soy, mercury (typically in fish) and dairy products. Eliminate them, and I am much better; introduce them into my diet, and irregular heartbeats result.

DELAY BETWEEN THE CAUSE AND THE SYMPTOM

There is another matter that affects the testing of your sensitivities to certain foods and drinks, notably the curious delay that occurs between the intake of the particular food or drink and the manifestation of the irregular heartbeat. Sometimes the delay could be as much as a day or more. In other words, you can eat some chocolate on Monday afternoon and not have any palpitations until Tuesday afternoon. This can significantly make your own analysis more difficult. But, I must point this out so you do not assume that you have no sensitivity if you do not experience a symptom within a couple of minutes to a couple of hours of the food or drink intake.

MERCURY POISONING MAY BE AFFECTING YOUR HEART RHYTHM

Outside of the above, there is an even scarier thought with respect to the cause of heartbeat abnormalities. Many experts believe that excessive mercury lodged in your heart muscle contributes to the interference with your electrical conduction system.[3] In fact, as early as 1952, it was found that one of the properties in mercury (called *"calomel"*) enhanced the influence of *epinephrine* (adrenaline) in constricting arteries and causing high blood pressure and rapid heart rate (tachychardia) in children. Science has proven mercury's toxic action on a wide range of tissues, including those in the cardiovascular system. Researchers have found that mercury affects several aspects of cardiac function, including the ability of heart muscle to contract, the electrical conduction activity in the heart, and the function of regulators of cardiac activity. Mercury toxic subjects have demonstrated an increased occurrence of rapid heartbeat, irregular pulse, chest pains, heart palpitations, and high blood pressure. For this reason, be careful to stay away from substances that contain mercury.

You must understand that mercury is an incredibly toxic and dangerous substance. According to the National Science Foundation and Western Resource Advocates, a non-profit environmental law and policy organization, emissions from coal-fired power plants are the single largest human-caused source of mercury in the environment. Coal plants contribute approximately one-third of all human-caused mercury. Coal-burning power plants are the only major source of mercury pollution in the United States that is not regulated by the government. When coal is burned at a power plant, mercury is released from the smoke stack and is ultimately deposited on land and in our rivers, streams, and lakes. In the United States, coal-fired plants pump about 50 tons of mercury into the air each year!

According to the Environmental and Occupational Health Sciences Institute in New Jersey, most human exposure to mercury comes from eating contaminated fish. Mercury accumulates in fish in a severely toxic form known as methylmercury. Over 40 states have mercury advisories warning consumers not to eat fish caught in certain lakes, streams, and other water bodies.

The U.S. Environmental Protection Agency (EPA) estimates that as many as seven million adults and children are regularly eating mercury-contaminated fish at unsafe levels. Mercury exposure at toxic levels can cause damage to vision, coordination, nervous system and brain function in adults and children. In addition, fetuses are particularly vulnerable to mercury poisoning, which can inhibit development and cause severe birth defects. Women are advised against eating fish with elevated levels of mercury both before and during pregnancy. For adults, there is a strong link between excessive amounts of mercury that you have in your body and heart disease (including interference with the normal sinus rhythm of your heart), as well as Parkinson's disease, multiple sclerosis, and even Alzheimer's disease.

Sadly, seafood is just one of the most common sources of mercury exposure to which you may be exposed. If you are consuming fish contaminated with mercury then you are setting the stage for future health problems, not to mention arrhythmias, because most of the fish that you eat contain unsafe levels of mercury. Big fish such as albacore tuna, shark and swordfish can contain as much as 100 times more mercury in their tissue than smaller fish.

Other Sources of Mercury Exposure

Another major source of mercury exposure is silver dental fillings. According to the International Academy of Oral Medicine and Toxicology, contrary to what many may assume, "silver" fillings are not entirely silver, for elemental mercury makes up half the substance of mercury fillings.

According to the World Health Organization and Dr. James Hardy in his book called *Mercury-Free*, studies have proven that people with mercury-containing dental fillings show a direct relationship between the number and size of the fillings and the amount of mercury found in their urine. Moreover, evidence has shown the level of mercury in the brain tissue of fetuses, newborns and young children is directly linked to the number of surface amalgam fillings the mother has. Mercury contamination is also an issue concerning pediatric vaccines. For decades, many people and infants, in particular, have injections of mercury though the thimerosal preservative used in such vaccines. In light of health dangers, the Food and Drug Administration recommended thimerosal be removed from all pediatric vaccines; it has been removed from all vaccines except for one – the influenza vaccine.

A Mercury Solution

So, let's say you have been eating fish for some time and are concerned with the level of toxic mercury within your cells. You have a toxic metals test and you are high in mercury. Well, the good news is that numerous studies in the USA and Europe indicate that chlorella, a form of green algae, is a powerful detoxification aid for heavy metals and other pesticides.[4] Chlorella can aid your body in the breakdown of persistent hydrocarbon and metallic toxins such as DDT, PCB, mercury, cadmium and lead, while strengthening your immune system. Chlorella can also aid the body in breaking down persistent hydrocarbon and metallic toxins such as mercury, cadmium and lead, DDT and PCB while strengthening the immune system response. In Japan, interest in chlorella has focused largely on its detoxifying properties – its ability to remove or neutralize poisonous substances from the body.

This detoxification of heavy metals and other chemical toxins in the blood will usually take 3 to 6 months to build up enough to begin this process depending on how much chlorella you are taking. And, since chlorella is a food, it is almost impossible to take too much chlorella.

Detoxification Properties

Chlorella is comprised of a fibrous, indigestible outer shell (20%) and its inner nutrients (80%). It is the fibrous material that has been proven to actually bind with the heavy metals and pesticides, such as PCBs, which can accumulate in your body. A clean bloodstream, with an abundance of red blood cells to carry oxygen, is necessary to a strong natural defense system. Chlorella's cleansing action on your bowel and other elimination channels, as well as its protection of your liver, helps keep your blood clean. Clean blood insures that your metabolic wastes are efficiently carried away from your tissues.

Chlorella gets its name from the high amount of chlorophyll it possesses. Chlorella contains more chlorophyll per gram than any other plant. Chlorophyll is one of the greatest food substances for cleansing the bowel and other elimination systems, such as the liver and the blood.

Green algae are the highest sources of chlorophyll in the plant world. And of all the green algae studied so far, chlorella has the highest, often ranging from 3 to 5% pure natural chlorophyll.

To summarize chapter 4, one of the most difficult diagnoses in medical science is that of irregular heartbeats in otherwise healthy individuals. It can result from the food you eat (and even love to eat), the beverages you consume or the prescription or non-prescription drugs you take. Every analysis becomes highly individualized, although the above is not as difficult as it might seem because there are some common denominators in terms of what causes irregular beats.

In order for you to determine the cause for your particular arrhythmia, you must be **proactive** in analyzing which chemical, foodstuff, and/or activity to which you might be sensitive. Finding the cause will be a slow experimental process. However, there is good news. The prevention suggestions in Chapter 5 can potentially suppress or even eliminate your symptoms so that the process of experimentation can be accomplished with less annoying side effects. Once you find the source, try to eliminate it from your life. If you cannot, then try to control it through implementing many of the suggestions you will find in Chapter 5.

Chapter 5
The Seven Natural & Safe Ways to Protect Against Irregular Heartbeats

"The art of medicine consists of amusing the patient while nature cures the disease."

—Voltaire

Well, this is what you have been waiting for – the seven natural and safe ways to protect against irregular heartbeats.

If one could invent the perfect formula to significantly reduce, prevent or even eliminate arrhythmias what would it look like? Well, the perfect formula would eliminate excessive irregular beats and do so with few side effects. And, it would do so without additional dangerous, life-threatening heart rhythms. This ideal anti-arrhythmia treatment would also help curb different kinds of arrhythmias (we only touched on a few of them, as there are several dozen varieties). In fact, it is not uncommon for a person to have both AFIB and ventricular arrhythmias, such as PVCs and PACs. Wouldn't a single effective agent for both disorders be nice? And, to even make this agent even more perfect, since we are dreaming up the perfect treatment, let's add something else – it would provide benefits that might even extend <u>beyond</u> arrhythmia correction. Is there any prescription medicine that comes close to our hypothetical remedy? Hardly!

However, there is a growing body of data and information (contained in numerous studies, reports, interviews, journals, periodicals and books) that strongly supports adopting certain nutritional approaches to reducing or keeping in check some rhythm disorders. While it may be indeed risky to try to treat your own arrhythmia, even with or without professional medical diagnosis based upon my personal experiences and the experiences of many of the cardiologists I have interviewed, a considerable degree of success can be achieved employing preventive nutritional and other "life-style change" strategies that may diminish the likelihood of future arrhythmias or lower the frequency and severity of an established rhythm disorder. Stated another way, I believe that natural strategies can really help you!

Throughout this book there are inferences that natural supplements can be more effective than prescription drugs, particularly from the standpoint of prevention. There are not only less harsh side effects of natural supplements than many heart related prescription drugs, but there is a plethora of beneficial side effects of the former. Notwithstanding, there are still some ground rules even when taking natural supplements.

First, if you are on prescription drugs, do some research on the interaction between such drugs and any natural supplements you may be taking to make sure that there are no known side effects. Some supplements can enhance the drugs, while others can interfere. Of course, the ultimate objective is to get off the drugs, but you must walk before you can run. Secondly, don't take supplements in the excess, as some of them can be just as harmful as prescription drugs if you take too much of them. Word to the wise – read the label and follow the instructions. Thirdly, be aware of the fact that certain vitamins, minerals and herbs work better with another supplement; so, be cognizant of this fact and research where this synergism between supplements may be applicable and try, where possible, to maximize the effect of the supplement without overusing it.

STRATEGY #1 – TAKE FISH OIL SUPPLEMENTS

If I were on a desert island and left with one supplement of my choice, that supplement would unequivocally be fish oil. Not only is fish oil inexpensive, safe, and effective, it is just about the best thing going in the quest for the perfect anti-arrhythmia supplement. And, this applies without mentioning fish oil's many, many other benefits that could very well be (and actually are) the subject of an entire book all to itself.

Fish oil is the most concentrated source of the omega-3 fatty acids (eicosopentaenoic acid (EPA) and docosapentaenoic acid (DHA)). Omega-3 fatty acids are very, very good for you and people do not take enough. In fact, for quite some time, omega-3 fatty acids have been recognized to play a key role in the prevention and treatment of cardiovascular-related diseases.[5] As reported in the July-

August 2000 issue of Nutrition, *Marine Oils: the Health Benefits of N-3 Fatty Acids*, fish oil powerfully inhibits the bodily processes that cause arrhythmias (see also Huggins, *Fish Oil May Reduce Irregular Heartbeat*, Circulation 2002;105). Fish oil not only sharply reduces the frequency of irregular beats, but it also diminishes the likelihood of death from dangerous arrhythmias. In fact, fish oil actually increases a desirable form of heart rate variability, as was discussed above at the beginning of this book. Most surprisingly, fish oil achieves all this without demonstrable side effects, something that every drug manufactured by the multi-billion dollar drug companies cannot claim with any degree of comfort.

Your heartbeat in and of itself is due to the electrical activity that results from small ions (sodium, calcium, and potassium) moving through specific pathways in the membrane of your heart's cells. Sometimes there will be mischievous cells that give off electrical activity independent of your heart's natural pacemaker (the SA node, if you recall). The omega-3 fatty acids eliminate the aberrational electrical activity from those problematical cells (that try to overwhelm your SA node's normal pace-making ability) by blocking excessive sodium and calcium currents in the channels of your heart. By regulating these two "ion" channels, omega-3 fatty acids preserve the normal electrical activity of your heart. And, the benefit takes place very quickly if you start consuming these fatty acids regularly.[6]

Fish oil's ability to curb arrhythmias are so effective that some insightful cardiologists are now recommending that patients with implanted defibrillators, which are used only for life-threatening heart rhythms, take fish oil to reduce their hearts' rhythm instability and to cut down on defibrillator firings, which are both painful and frightening.

As far as taking fish oil from a preventative standpoint, the Physician's Health Study noted above[7] concluded that, based on many years of examination, the people who died from sudden death had much lower levels of omega-3 fatty acids than those who did not. Just eating one or more servings of fish weekly resulted in a sizeable 52% reduction in the risk of sudden death.

Now, compare omega-3 fatty acids with a substance known as *"arachidonic acid"*, which results from your intake of the bad omega-6 fatty acids. These omega-6 fatty acids actually have the opposite effect from omega-3 fatty acids. In other words, the omega-6 fatty acids increase your potential for arrhythmias! So, the logical conclusion is to learn about what you eat that contains an excessive amount of omega-6 fatty acids and reduce or eliminate these foods. And, increase your intake of omega-3 fatty acids. I will discuss omega-6 fatty acids in more detail on the next few pages and in Part II of this book.

Another heart related benefit of fish oil is that it reduces the blood clotting protein called fibrinogen. This reduces the risk of blood clot formation on coronary plaque that could very easily result in a heart attack.[8]

Fish Oil and AFIB

Probably, one of the most interesting questions is whether fish oil can actually curb AFIB (that is, AFIB resulting from any cause). As stated in Chapter 3, with AFIB you are not having blood pumped out of your atria effectively, and your blood can pool and clot, increasing the risk for stroke. Conventional medical treatment for AFIB is fraught with side effects and is of limited effectiveness, and better therapies are clearly needed.[9] One study undertaken a few years ago concluded that fish oil impressively suppressed AFIB in experimental non-human preparations.[10] Another study in 2004 concluded that people who suffer from AFIB have demonstrably lower levels of omega-3 fatty acids.[11] Well, I doubt that the modern medical community would whole-heartedly (no pun intended) embrace fish oil as the "cure all" remedy. From an utterly selfish standpoint, many years will pass before cardiologists recognize something as simple as fish oil will be a primary mechanism to suppress AFIB. Remember, from time to time the drug companies pay the doctors financial incentives to prescribe expensive drug medications; and you pay a doctor good money for office consultations, to largely prescribe drugs.

The evidence is quite compelling and it is very difficult not to conclude that fish oil is the most effective non-prescription drug agent in the world for suppressing heart arrhythmias, particularly PCs and AFIB.

So, the issue is, do you unhesitatingly start to increase your fish consumption immediately? Read on!

The Other Ancillary Benefits of Fish Oil

Obviously, this book is not intended to be a full-scale analysis of the benefits of fish oil. But, I absolutely cannot discuss the benefits of fish oil for your heart without talking about the enormous benefits for your entire well-being. To a certain extent, comparing the benefits of fish oil with any of the modern anti-arrhythmia medicines is like comparing apples and.... (not oranges) but an entire orange grove, blueberry farm, strawberry patch...all combined. In other words, there is no comparison.

You want to increase your overall health and energy level. You want to help in preventing cancer, depression and Alzheimer's? Perhaps you also want to address or reduce the symptoms of rheumatoid arthritis, diabetes, ulcerative colitis, Raynaud's disease and a host of other diseases? Or, maybe you don't have any of these diseases, but just want to lose weight (by processing body fat more efficiently), increase daily energy levels and/or have healthier, younger-looking skin. Maybe you are pregnant and want to avoid premature birth and low birth weight. One of the most important things you can do to assist in achieving all of these benefits is to increase your intake of the omega-3 fats found in fish oil and cod liver oil, and reduce your intake of omega-6 fats.

Omega-3 and Omega-6 Fatty Acids

These two types of fatty acids, omega-3 and omega-6, are both essential for human health. However, the typical American consumes far too many omega-6 fats in their diet while consuming very low levels of omega-3. The ideal ratio of omega-6 to omega-3 fats is 1:1. Our ancestors evolved over millions of years on this ratio. Today, though, our ratio of omega-6 to omega-3 averages from 20:1 to 50:1! That means it's very dangerous for you, and as is now finally being reported throughout even the mainstream health media, lack of omega-3 from fish oil is one of the most serious health issues plaguing contemporary society.

The primary sources of omega-6 are corn, soy, canola, safflower and sunflower oil; these oils are overabundant in the typical diet, which explains our excess omega-6 levels. Avoid or limit these oils for this reason and for many other reasons discussed below. Omega-3, meanwhile, is typically found in flaxseed oil, walnut oil, and fish.

The use of flaxseed oil is interesting. Another type of fatty acid called alpha-linolenic acid (ALA) is found in flaxseed oil, walnuts and canola oil. However, when humans ingest ALA only 10% of it is converted into active EPA and DHA, while most of the rest is burned for calories. Anecdotally, I must point out that according to Dr. Charles Myers at the University of Virginia Medical School, there is evidence indicating that flax seed oil may promote the growth of prostate tumors. Thus, if you have prostate cancer you should avoid flax seed oil and instead take 2-3 grams per day of fish oil.

By far, the best type of omega-3 fat is that found in fish. That's because the omega-3 in fish is high in two fatty acids crucial to human health, DHA and EPA. These two fatty acids are pivotal in helping to prevent heart disease, cancer, and many other diseases. Your human brain is also highly dependent on DHA –

low DHA levels have been linked to depression, schizophrenia, memory loss, and a higher chance of developing Alzheimer's.

Most of the empirical data shows that fish oil capsules providing a daily dose of 1000-2000 mg of EPA and DHA have remarkable and significant benefits.

The Dangers of Eating Fresh Fish

If you think that you can simply eat more fish, you are sadly mistaken. Eating most fresh fish, whether from the ocean, lakes and streams, or farm-raised, is no longer recommended. Mercury levels in almost all fish have now hit very high levels across the globe, and the risk of this mercury to your health now outweighs the fish's omega-3 benefits.

As I alluded to above, with respect to the causation of irregular heartbeats, mercury, a poisonous substance, is lodged in the fish you eat. What has happened is that the combustion in power plants of coal containing mercury is the major source of environmental pollution. Many, many tons of mercury is released into the U.S. every year by this method through pollution and waste. Mercury pollution from coal-fired power plants moves through the environment and can transform into organic mercury, which is known as methylmercury, and accumulate in steams, oceans, water and soil. Methylmercury also accumulates in the sea creatures underwater, so each fish absorbs the mercury in other fish and the organisms it eats. For this reason, larger and older fish such as fresh shark, tuna and swordfish contain the highest levels of methylmercury. Every effort should be made to avoid these fish, plain and simple.

Fish like tuna, sea bass, marlin and halibut also show some of the worst contamination, but dozens of species and thousands of water bodies have been seriously polluted.

People who regularly eat fish have higher levels of methylmercury than those who do not. Also, methylmercury can harm a developing baby's brain and nervous system. Consequently, pregnant or breastfeeding women who eat a lot of fish put their newborns at risk. Other groups that are particularly sensitive to mercury exposure include children under the age of 6 years, people with impaired kidney function and people with sensitive immune responses to metals.

Methylmercury toxicity can result in a condition known as *paraesthesia* (a tingling sensation on the skin), depression, and blurred vision. In fetuses and developing infants methylmercury can also have negative effects on attention span, language, visual-spatial skills, memory and coordination. Scientists estimate that nearly 60,000 children each year are born at risk for neurological problems due to methylmercury exposure in the womb.

Both the Food and Drug Administration (FDA) and the Environmental Protection Agency (EPA) have issued health advisories about consuming fish due to methylmercury contamination. The FDA recommends that pregnant women, nursing mothers and children limit their consumption of fish to 12 ounces per week and completely avoid shark, swordfish, king mackerel and tilefish (also known as golden bass and golden snapper). The EPA has issued even stricter guidelines.

Since Americans consume so much of tuna, particular concern has been raised about this fish. Canned tuna typically has lower levels of methylmercury than fresh tuna because canned tuna usually comes from smaller fish. However, since Americans eat canned tuna in high quantities, eating it could still pose a risk. The FDA recommends that pregnant women, nursing mothers and children limit their consumption of tuna to no more than one 6-ounce can per week, as it is possible that more could result in neurological damages to babies and young children.

Some of the less harmful fish/seafood include catfish, blue crab, tilapia, croaker, fish sticks, flounder, haddock, trout (farmed), salmon (wild Pacific and Alaskan) and shrimp. The fish to limit and to otherwise be very careful of include canned tuna, sea bass, oysters, marlin, halibut, pike, walleye, largemouth bass, mahi mahi, cod, pollack, lake whitefish, and Great Lakes salmon.

There is a website called www.gotmercury.org, that actually calculates the amount of mercury exposure for you based upon your fish intake per portion and over an extended period of time. It is not foolproof, but quite helpful.

Farm Raised vs. Wild Salmon

I have one final note on fish and that has to do with salmon. This species is probably the one with the highest degree of the good omega-3 oil on the planet, not to mention good, fresh salmon tastes heavenly. Much of the salmon that you see in the traditional grocery stores and most restaurants are farm raised salmon. Succinctly stated, stay away from this type of salmon in most cases. While fresh Alaskan or Pacific salmon may be one of the healthiest foods on the planet, paradoxically, most (although not necessarily all) farm-raised salmon may be one the worst foods on the planet!

Unfortunately, nearly all farmed salmon have the same mercury problem, but have much higher amounts of toxic pollutants, such as PCBs and dioxins and have much lower amounts of beneficial omega-3 than wild-caught salmon. Notably, dioxins are released when industrial waste is burned, and PCBs was once widely used as insulating material (see box below). Farm raised Atlantic salmon are farmed in large-scale, densely stocked netpen facilities. Fish often escape, and can compete for resources, breed with, or spread parasites to wild fish. Salmon farms often allow feces, excess feed, and any chemicals used to flow freely into surrounding waters.

Dioxins and PCBs in Fish and Shellfish

According to the non-profit Environmental Defense Network, dioxins are highly toxic byproducts of industrial processes. Like many other contaminants found in fish, these chemicals are slow to break down, and they accumulate in the bottom sediments of streams, rivers, lakes and coastal areas. Dioxins can build up in the fatty tissues of fish and other animals, and in high enough concentrations pose serious health risks to people who frequently eat contaminated fish.

Small amounts of dioxins are produced naturally during forest fires and volcanic eruptions. However, the majority of dioxins in the environment are an unwanted result of human industrial processes, such as the production of certain herbicides and disinfectants, waste incineration, and chlorine bleaching of pulp at paper mills. Improved pollution controls and changes in manufacturing processes have in some instances reduced releases of dioxins to the environment. According to pamphlets and fact sheets issued by the National Institute of Environmental Health Sciences, studies conducted on laboratory animals resulted in the conclusion that dioxins increase your cancer risk and can harm your immune system. Effects on reproductive, endocrine, circulatory and nervous systems have also been observed. TCDD (the most hazardous of the dioxin compounds) exhibits the highest cancer potency of any chemical ever studied in animals.

PCBs, or polychlorinated biphenyls, are highly toxic man-made industrial compounds. They pose serious health risks to fetuses, babies and children, who may suffer developmental and neurological problems from prolonged or repeated exposure to small amounts of PCBs. These chemicals are harmful to adults as well. Although they were banned from manufacture in the United States in 1977, PCBs are slow to break down and can persist in the environment at dangerous levels. PCBs accumulate in the sediments at the bottoms of streams, rivers, lakes and coastal areas. These chemicals can build up in the fatty tissues of fish and other animals, and in high concentrations pose serious health risks to people who frequently eat contaminated fish.

A combination of useful chemical properties made PCBs popular for a variety of industrial applications, including use in electrical transformers, hydraulic fluids, lubricants and carbonless paper. More than 1.5 billion pounds of PCBs were manufactured in the United States before they were banned, and some electrical equipment in use today still contains PCBs.

Unfortunately, the same properties that made PCBs ideal for industrial use make them slow to break down in the environment. Most PCBs do not mix with water and settle into riverbeds, lake bottoms and coastal sediments. Here they can enter the food chain and bio-accumulate in invertebrates, fish, birds and mammals – including people. Although these chemicals have been banned for many years, increased testing has recently shown that the problem of PCB-contaminated fish is widespread.

Wild salmon eat creatures like shrimp and krill, which contain chemicals that make salmon pink. Since farm-raised fish do not eat a natural diet, their flesh would be gray if not for artificial additives. The chemicals used to turn farm-raised fish pink (canthaxanthin and astaxanthin) make them more marketable, since many consumers prefer fish with the traditional pink color. However, there is "significant controversy" over the effects of canthaxanthin, as it has been associated with retinal damage in the human eye.

Interestingly, many salmon farmers in the United States, Canada and Chile are slowly replacing some of the fish oil in salmon feed with soybean and canola oil to address the contaminants. Ironically, that may correct the pollutants per se, but the change does not address the lowering of the beneficial omega-3 fatty acid by infusing the fish with the more harmful omega-6 fatty acid, which is so prevalent in soybean and canola oil!

Now, having stated all that, there are some commercial farms located in certain parts of the world where precautions are taken to make sure that the fish are fed a more natural diet and that their waters are well managed. Retailers of these farm-raised fish are highly selective about what they sell, and dedicated to stringent quality standards, and committed to sustainable agriculture. It is therefore important to ask your seafood vendor lots of questions, even though he or she might not know all the answers, the more you ask, the more the vendor will recognize the need to provide better information about sourcing and fishing practices. Based upon my experience, an example of a major national retailer of quality farm-raised salmon and other fish products is the Whole Foods Market, based in Austin, Texas.

And, the situation doesn't get any better, either. A study conducted in early 2005 by Canadian researchers determined that even wild baby salmon that pass commercial salmon farms on their way to the ocean are being infected with sea lice at rates 73 times higher than normal. Such parasites feed off the skin, blood and flesh of these baby fish, killing them early in their development. Antibiotics control the spread of these sea lice within fish farms, but these young fish (actually, they are called "smolts") passing through these farms to the ocean have no safeguard.

The point of this story is that we are continually facing threats to our supply of fresh, disease free seafood. And, the situation seems to be getting worse rather than better. Either you have fish infected with sea lice or you are eating fish that are treated with antibiotics – an agent that keeps the fish alive so that it can injure the life of yourself and other seafood lovers. This is just one more example of how biotechnology has transformed fish, in the past one of the most nutritious foods you could eat, into an unhealthy food – especially if you purchase the fish at a traditional grocery store or restaurant.

STRATEGY #2 – MILK THAT MAGNESIUM

Magnesium is a crucial nutrient that helps ensure the proper functioning of approximately 300 enzymes in the human body. Unfortunately, magnesium is one of the most underused minerals by mankind. The average American ingests substantially less than the daily recommended dietary allowance (RDA) of 420 mg of magnesium for men and 320 mg for women.

Researchers are becoming more aware of the fact that magnesium intake is dropping considerably and have concluded that Americans are consuming more and more magnesium depleted foods. Soft drinks, for example, are manufactured with de-ionized water and are essentially devoid of magnesium. Carbonated beverages like soda contain phosphates, making magnesium unavailable for absorption in your intestinal tract. To make matters worse, more and more people are drinking bottled water, and most retail brands contain little or no magnesium.

Even tap water is getting into the act. Municipal and home water treatment systems convert hard water into soft water, thus removing the magnesium. Interestingly, demonstrable increases in the risk of sudden death have been reported in cities with the lowest level of magnesium in their drinking water. In fact, a recent World Health Organization report on the quality of drinking water cited a number of studies that examined the relationship between cardiovascular death and water "hardness" (measured principally by magnesium and calcium content). The report concluded that the magnesium content of water is indeed a heart health risk and should become a priority for water supplementation.

In hospitals where blood levels are frequently monitored, when magnesium blood levels are low, arrhythmias tend to occur. These arrhythmias run the gamut of variability, from premature or irregular nuisance rhythms all the way to dangerous rhythms. People suffering from congestive heart failure are especially susceptible to these rhythms when magnesium levels are low. People prone to AFIB are more prone to have recurrences due to low magnesium levels.

The bad news is that measuring your magnesium levels is not easy. You know those blood tests you take at your annual physical. Granted, they are supposed to measure your blood magnesium levels. However, even if blood levels of magnesium are normal, you may still have low tissue levels of magnesium. And, you guessed it, just about the first place where there is a glaring reduction in tissue magnesium is in the heart muscle!

So, how do you know if your magnesium level is too low? Well, if you have any sort of arrhythmia, you should question whether or not you have adequate levels of magnesium since low magnesium levels tend to trigger abnormal heart rhythms. Low potassium also accompanies low magnesium. Nightly leg cramps (when you are not doing any walking) is also an indicator of low magnesium. Additional symptons include tremors, anxiety and weakness.

While the treatment of specific abnormal heart rhythms is normally reserved for your physician or cardiologist, ensuring sufficient magnesium intake is an excellent preventative strategy that is strongly supported by the scientific literature. Optimal magnesium levels tend to make all sorts of problemmatical rhythms, including PVCs, PACs and AFIB being less likely to occur. Although some have argued that magnesium administered during acute heart attack does not reduce the risk of dying from fatal heart arrhythmias, magnesium can be very effective in less dire situations.

Because low magnesium tissue levels are commonplace in America and in most countries, magnesium supplementation should be undertaken by nearly everyone. Many epidemiologists (for your technical information, this is a person, usually a medical doctor, who deals with the study of the causes, distribution, and control of disease in populations) have proposed supplementing tap water with magnesium, just as floride is added to prevent tooth decay. Magnesium supplements are safe and inexpensive, and the only side effects are increased bowel movements (which is not a bad thing at all) and loose stools, or in the extreme case, diarrhea. This can occur in doses which are as little as 250 mg. although the average tolerable amount is much higher.

For magnesium supplememtation, the mainstream medical doctor's typical recommeded dose is from 300-500 mg. daily. However, the better choice is to take as much as 1500 mg. of magnesium in distributed doses throughout the day. This is because some people have different metabolisms than others. Take as much as you can giving due regard to the amount of magnesium included in any multi-vitamin you take. If your stool becomes too loose, simply cut back. You will eventually reach the right daily amount. The rule of thumb, without being too graphic, is to take as much as you can so that you can actually have a loose stool, but not diarrhea per se. If your bowel movements increase from 1 per day to 2 or 3 per day, don't be alarmed – this means that things are working.

Good dietary sources of magnesium can be found in barley, oat bran (that's why you may sometimes hear that oat bran muffins are good for your heart), pumpkin seeds, trail mix, soybeans, spinach, and whole grain wheat flour, just to name a few.

STRATEGY #3 – STRENGTHEN YOUR HEART AND WEAKEN YOUR ARRHYTHMIA WITH COENZYME Q10

Coenzyme Q10 (CoQ10 for short) is a powerhouse of a nutrient. CoQ10 is found in that part of your body's cells that generate energy (which is called the *mitochondria*). CoQ10 has been shown to be able to stabilize your cell membranes, a feature that might have the potential for influencing heart rhythms.[12]

So, let's examine what happens when there there is a heart problem and see what happens to your heart muscle. Many arrhythmias occur when there is abnormal weakness of your heart muscle, a viral infection of your heart, or abnormal thickening of your heart muscle (the latter of which is common in people with high blood pressure). These situations are irritating to your heart and make it electrically unstable. An arrhythmia can result.

Study after study shows that CoQ10 supplementation can benefit you if you have a weakened heart muscle. Now, these studies primarily focus on situations where there is heart disease present, rather than address the healthy person that simply has troublesome irregular beats. But, the fact is that CoQ10 produces substantial improvements in palpitations in these patients. Overall, the data is consistent in showing the people feel and breathe better, suffer less build up of fluid in the legs, experience fewer palpitations, and are able to exercise longer when taking CoQ10.[13] CoQ10 is also effective in reducing blood pressure. As you may have experienced, elevated blood pressure typically accompanies PCs and AFIB.[14] Well, high blood pressure and its associated thickened heart muscle underlie several varieties of abnormal heart rhythms, especially atrial fibrillation.

CoQ10 also reduces angina attacks, congestive heart failure, periodontal disease, and heart valve irregularities; it is protective to smokers; and supplies energy to the heart.

So, does CoQ10 reduce abnormal rhythms? While that specific question is hard to categorically answer in the affirmative, there have been studies conducted that tend to show that after administering CoQ10, there is a dramatic drop in abnormal heart rhythms when recovering from a heart attack, or while having high blood pressure or suffering diabetes.

As to whether this relates to a healthier heart for you, notably if you have occasional PCs or AFIB, one thing is for certain. CoQ10 is a safe, effective nutritional agent that is virtually free of side effects. It may certainly help lessen the long term risk of arrhythmias through its actions in substantially lowering blood pressure and increasing left ventricular muscle strength. Whether CoQ10 has a direct action in reducing arrhythmias or whether it simply helps correct the underlying conditions that lead to arrhythmias is still not clear. It is just an excellent preventative supplement to lessen the likelihood of developing irregular heartbeats.

What dosage of CoQ10 is best? Most studies and recommended dosages on bottles of the product seem to focus around 50-150 mg as being that which has an impact. Much greater amounts are prescribed for serious heart trouble. Without ascribing to the theory of "more is better" it seems that 200-250 mg per day is optimum to effectively contribute to your anti-arrhythmia regimen.

STRATEGY #4 – NATTOKINASE: THE "WONDER" ALTERNATIVE TO ASPIRIN AND BLOOD THINNING DRUGS

A truly revolutionary powerful enzyme called nattokinase, derived from a food called natto, has been used by the Japanese for years. This plant has produced monumental success for dissolving blood clots.[15]

How Blood Clots Form

You now know, from the information contained in Chapters 2 and 3, about the risk of blood clots forming. Blood clots (also known as *thrombi*) form when strands of protein called fibrin accumulate in one of your blood vessels. In your heart, blood clots cause blockage of blood flow to muscle tissue. If blood flow is blocked, the oxygen supply to that tissue is cut off and the heart tissue eventually dies. This can result in a condition known as angina (which is a heart condition marked by sudden, not to mention intense, attacks of chest pain due to reduced oxygen to the heart) and heart attacks. Clots in chambers of your heart can mobilize to your brain. In your brain, blood clots also block blood and oxygen from reaching necessary areas, which can result in your becoming senile and/or having stroke.

There are enzymes in your body that break up blood clots. These enzymes, known as *thrombolytic enzymes,* are normally generated in certain of your blood cells. These are the *endothelial cells* of your blood vessels. Sadly, as your body ages, production of these enzymes begins to decline, making your blood more prone to coagulation. This mechanism can lead to heart problems or stroke noted above, as well as other conditions. Once your endothelial cells start to produce less thrombolytic enzymes this affects your whole body since your endothelial cells exist everywhere throughout your body, such as in your arteries, veins and lymphatic system. This means that poor production of thrombolytic enzymes can lead to the development of blood clot conducive conditions virtually anywhere in your body.

Thrombotic diseases, which are diseases from blood clots, typically include bleeding in the brain area (cerebral hemorrhage), cells dying in your brain or heart resulting from the obstruction of blood supply (which is called cerebral and cardiac infarction, respectively) and angina pectoris. The term, thrombotic diseases, can also include diseases caused by blood vessels with lowered flexibility, including senile dementia and diabetes (caused by your pancreas failing due to lack of proper blood supply).

Recent studies have revealed that the clogging of the blood vessels in your brain due to blood clotting may be a cause of dementia. A somewhat shocking, although not totally surprising, statistic is that in Japan, researchers estimate that sixty percent of senile dementia patients in Japan is caused by blood clots in brain cells.

Hemorrhoids are considered a more localized, less dangerous condition of blood clotting. And, all this does not include chronic diseases of the capillaries. If they are taken into consideration, then the number of blood clot related conditions may be much higher.

Nattokinase does more than prevent clots from forming. It re-activates your own natural blood thinning stores of an enzyme called *urokinase* to levels that existed when you were years younger. Nattokinase effectively dissolves and breaks down the protein that causes clotting, called *fibrin* strands. When these strands are removed from your blood, your flow improves and your cells are revitalized with a greater degree of oxygen. With less blood thickness, there is less blood viscosity or resistance and this strikes at the root of atherosclerosis (a common disorder of the arteries where fat, cholesterol, and other substances accumulate in the walls of your arteries and form plaques). These plaques that rupture cause blood clots to form that can block blood flow or break off and travel to another part of your body. If either happens and blocks a blood vessel that feeds the heart, it causes a heart attack. If it blocks a blood vessel that feeds the brain, it causes a stroke.

Nattokinase has been used safely for over 20 years, and unlike aspirin, has not been known to produce any negative side effects – and it is not known to be an allergen. Nattokinase is a convenient, consistent, and powerful prevention mechanism as well as an agent that can provide support if you have inherent heart weaknesses.

Other Benefits of Nattokinase

The Japanese have long believed that consuming natto regularly leads to lower blood pressure.[16] Over the past several years, several clinical trials have substantiated their claim. In a 1995 study, researchers confirmed the presence of ACE inhibitors in natto (ACE inhibitors are good and you will learn more about them latter in my discussion about blood pressure).[17] Now, there is a very potent chemical in your body that causes the muscles surrounding your blood vessels to contract, which in turn causes your blood vessel pathways to narrow (this chemical is called *angiotensin II*). The narrowing of the vessels increases the pressure within the vessels and can cause high blood pressure (hypertension). *Angiotensin II* is formed from angiotensin I in the blood by the enzyme called *angiotensin converting enzyme* (ACE). ACE inhibitors are medications that slow (inhibit) the activity of the enzyme, which decreases the production of *angiotensin II*. As a result, the blood vessels enlarge or dilate, and the blood pressure is reduced. This lower blood pressure makes it easier for the heart to pump blood.

Among its many other remarkable properties, nattokinase has shown the ability to:

- prevent heart attacks and strokes
- decrease blood thickness allowing improved blood flow and circulation
- increase oxygen deliverability (energy)
- increase the availability of other nutrients and supplements
- decrease blood pressure, both systolic and diastolic
- decrease the risk of deep vein thrombosis (DVT) (where blood clots clog one of the major deep veins of your arms, lower legs, thighs or pelvis and frequently resulting from long air travel)

Other benefits abound with nattokinase, such as:

- decreased varicose veins
- improved vision
- improved bone density
- minimized joint pain in osteoarthritis and rheumatoid arthritis
- reduction of migraine headaches
- decreased cholesterol
- prevention of joint and muscles pains from excessive physical exertion

This remarkable enzyme can also improve digestion and promote longevity. Under good conditions, natto bacteria can double in 30 minutes, producing various enzymes that help digestion – breaking down soybean nutrients that are difficult for humans to digest. These enzymes include *protease* that breaks down protein into amino acids; *amylase* that converts complex carbohydrates into glucose; lipase breaks down neutral fat into glycerin and fatty acids; *cellulase* breaks down fibers into simpler carbohydrates.

The difference with nattokinasse is that most of the bacteria beneficial to your intestines such as *bifidus* are killed in your stomach by the acid before they reach your intestines if taken orally. But natto bacteria are able to survive the journey and reproduce in your intestines where they aid digestion.

Some progressive physicians are also looking at nattokinase as an anti-aging enzyme (most mainstream physicians, including cardiologists, don't even know of its existence). Because fibrin accumulation can eventually interfere with oxygen and nutrient transfer to your body's cells and removal of waste products, fibrin hampers the primary functions of your blood – a critical factor in aging. And, as an additional byproduct, is a good source of protein and vitamin B2, which keeps your skin young.

Where Does Nattokinase Come From

Natto is a traditional Japanese food and is commonly eaten for breakfast in Japan. Since natto is made from soybeans fermented by natto bacillus, it is sticky and has strong smell and taste. Nattokinase is currently produced by a fermentation process by adding bacillus natto, a beneficial type of bacteria, to boiled soybeans. Natto has slippery-sticky paste on its surface, and once stirred, the slippery paste increases in volume forming spider web-like threads. Because of its somewhat unpleasant odor, some people dislike eating natto, although fans of bleu cheese will probably love natto. Others will happily appreciate the capsule form. But, natto is known as a nutritious food in Japan, and the popularity has been increasing in recent years.

For centuries, however, natto was easily made at home; soybeans were packed in straw (which contained a natural bacillus) then buried for a week in the ground. Today, natto is made by injecting the bacteria. The bacillus natto acts on the soybeans, producing the nattokinase enzyme. Other soy foods contain enzymes, but only the natto preparation contains the specific nattokinase enzyme. When compared to ordinary soybeans, the natto produces more calories, fiber, calcium, potassium and B2. Natto has slightly less protein than beef, but contains more fiber, iron and nearly double the calcium and vitamin E.

How Was Nattokinase Discovered

As noted above, natto has been a traditional Japanese food for more than 1,000 years. According to Japanese folklore, the famous warrior Yoshiie Minamoto was responsible for introducing natto to northwestern Japan. Ancient Samurai warriors consumed natto on a daily basis and even fed it to their horses to increase their speed and strength. During the Edo Period (1603–1867), natto was given to pregnant women to insure a healthy newborn. In other words, the Japanese use natto extensively and now you can understand why the Japanese, despite other cultural foibles from a health and nutrition standpoint, have fared quite well in combating heart disease.

In 1928, Dr. Alexander Fleming, after examining some colonies of staph bacteria, noted that a mold called *penicillium notatum* had formed. The mold prevented the normal growth of the staphylococci. Dr. Fleming realized that something in the penicillium mold inhibited the growth of the bacteria – and even more importantly – that it might also be harnessed in creating medicines to combat infectious diseases that were killing with a vengeance.

Similarly, the real discovery of nattokinase (as applied to blood thinning) is generally credited to Dr. Hiroyuki Sumi in 1980 while working as a researcher at the University of Chicago. Dr. Sumi had long researched thrombolytic enzymes searching for a natural agent that could successfully dissolve thrombus associated with blood clots associated with heart attacks and stroke (technically called "cardiac and cerebral infarction"). Sumi discovered nattokinase in 1980 while working as a researcher and majoring in physiological chemistry at Chicago University Medical School. After testing over 173 natural foods as potential thrombolytic agents, Sumi found what he was looking for when Natto was dropped onto a blood clot in an experimental dish and allowed it to stand at 37 degrees centigrade (approximately body temperature). The blood clot (again, they call this a "thrombus" if you crave medical techno terms) around the natto dissolved gradually and had completely dissolved within 18 hours. Sumi named the newly discovered enzyme "nattokinase", which means "enzyme in natto". Sumi commented that nattokinase showed "a potency matched by no other enzyme."[18]

How Nattokinase is Different

So, why does nattokinasse work where other medicines fail? Your body contains several enzymes that actually promote the formation of blood clots, but it produces only one enzyme, which is called plasmin that actually dissolves them.

Unfortunately, as you would expect, like many other beneficial enzymes, plasmin diminishes as we grow older. The properties of nattokinase closely resemble those of plasmin and are able to dissolve fibrin directly while enhancing your body's natural production of both plasmin and other clot dissolving agents.

Conventional medicine, notably the drug companies, has created several drugs that are supposed to dissolve blood clots. The medical community calls these drugs "tissue plasminogen activactors" (t-PAs). By name they have such names as *actiase, urokinase and streptokinase*. Every year, stroke and heart attack victims are given these drugs and, recognizably, they do save hundreds of thousands of lives.

But, not surprisingly, these drugs are very expensive. Nattokinase, by comparison, is much less expensive by a wide margin when compared to the blood thinning drugs manufactured by our profit mongering, multi-billion dollar drug companies. For example, one dose of urokinase costs approximately $1,500! However, nattokinase is comparable to the cost of quality vitamins. For example, a typical preventative dose is about 100 mg (also expressed in fibrin units, which would be around 1800). This normally would cost less than a dollar a day! Of course, for individuals with a history of heart trouble, the dosage, according to the manufacturers that make it, is two or three times as much.

Not only are the prescription drugs expensive, they don't last long. Urokinase starts to lose its impact as rapidly as 4-20 minutes after administration, while nattokinase keeps the blood clear for 4 to 8 hours – significantly impacting the ability to achieve a full recovery from heart attacks and strokes!

Also, you have to take the drugs through an IV; however, drugs often fail when your arteries have hardened beyond the point where the dissolving agent can treat them. The key here is the prevention of the hardening of the arteries in the first place and that is where nattokinase comes into play. Nattokinase is unique in that it complements your body's protection against inadvertent blood clots without impairing your body's ability to quickly form clots to prevent bleeding from a cut, and essentially stopping excess blood loss after a trauma. While pharmaceutical agents inhibit this critical coagulation process in hopes of preventing a blood clot, nattokinase will not.

The Controversy Surrounding Soy Products

You might wonder about the safety of natto, since it is a derivative of soy, particularly since there has been a considerable amount of controversy surrounding the safety of consuming soy products.

If you have been reading about soy lately, you probably have been second guessing the benefits that mainstream nutritionists and food purveyors have been spoon feeding the American public for years. Traditionally, soy has been viewed as an excellent source of protein, not to mention lowering cholesterol, protecting against cancer and heart disease, reducing menopause symptoms, and preventing osteoporosis, among other things. However, if you do some research on the subject you will find the real reason why there's so much soy in America.

When the soy industry got started, soy was planted for the purpose of extracting the oil from it. However, according to Dr. Kaayla Daniel, author of the book *The Whole Soy Story: The Dark Side of America's Favorite Health Food*, today's high-tech processing methods not only fail to remove the anti-nutrients and toxins that are naturally present in soybeans but leave toxic and carcinogenic residues created by the high temperatures, high pressure, alkali and acid baths and petroleum solvents. The worst of today's soy protein products are soy protein isolate, soy protein concentrate, texturized vegetable protein and hydrolyzed vegetable protein. These ingredients are in everything from shake powders, energy bars and veggie burgers to canned tuna. The worst soy oil products are margarines and shortenings made from partially hydrogenated soybean oil containing dangerous trans fatty acids (read more on trans fatty acids in chapter 8 of this book). Many of the liquid vegetable oils sold in food stores also come from the soybean. To make these oils palatable enough for the general public to accept, they are subjected to heavy refining, deodorizing and light hydrogenation.

So, how did soy, once a fringe product, end up being thought of as a "disease-preventive panacea"? According to Daniel, for years, the market for soy foods was limited. Americans did not like the "beany" taste and gas-producing effects of soy and viewed soy products as something for vegetarians. That presented a problem to the industry, which had lots of soy protein left over from soy oil production and nowhere to sell it. After all, they could only feed so much to animals before they came down with serious health problems. In order to make a good profit selling soy protein as a "people feed," the industry needed to make people want to eat it and to pay well for the privilege.

A marketing executive for the soy industry explained three decades ago, "the quickest way to gain product acceptability in the less affluent society is to have the product consumed on its own merit by a more affluent society." Increased consumer awareness of the "health benefits" of soy did its job. Millions of soy industry dollars were funneled into medical research, sponsoring symposia, establishing FDA health claims and influencing of key dietitians and journalists. The campaign led to a lot of soy propaganda, high hopes and higher profits.

Soybean oil ultimately became a very large industry. Once the soybean producers incorporated soybean oil as they did in the food supply, they had a lot of soy protein residue left over. And, since they cannot feed it to animals, except in small amounts, they had to find another market.

This other market was a health and wellness foodstuff. The industry spent millions of dollars on advertising and intensely lobbied to the Food and Drug Administration (FDA). So now, most American consumers believe soy products are healthy.

However, notions of objectivity and reality suggest a different conclusion. To illustrate, consider that numerous studies have found that soy products may (i) increase the risk of breast cancer in women, brain damage in both men and women, and abnormalities in infants, (ii) contribute to thyroid disorders, especially in women, (iii) e, (iv) weaken the immune system, and (v) cause severe, potentially fatal food allergies.[19] Soy products also contain certain chemicals which (i) mimic and sometimes block the hormone estrogen (called *phytoestrogens* (isoflavones) genistein and daidzein), (ii) which block your body's uptake of minerals (called *phytates*), (iii) which hinder your protein digestion) (called *enzyme inhibitors*) and (iv) which cause your red blood cells to clump together and inhibit oxygen take-up and growth (called *haemaggluttin*).[20]

Sounds like pretty technical terms, but there is one thing that is easy to understand – soy isn't what it is cracked up to be by big business executives whose main objective is to generate profits for their corporations, and ironically place health and wellness as a secondary goal. When you consider that two-thirds of all manufactured food products contain some form of soy (according to the Institute of Food Research (IFR), a not-for-profit company sponsored by the Biotechnology & Biological Sciences Research Council), it becomes clear just how many Americans are consuming these products, whose long-term effects are completely unknown.[21]

Perhaps the most disturbing of soy's problematical effects on health involves its *phytoestrogens* that can mimic the effects of the female hormone estrogen. These *phytoestrogens* have been found to have adverse effects on various human tissues, and drinking even two glasses of soymilk daily for one month has enough of the chemical to alter your menstrual cycle if you are a woman. The FDA regulates estrogen-containing products; however, no warnings exist on soy. Two senior toxicologists with the FDA, Daniel Sheehan and Daniel Doerge, have even come out saying "the public will be put at potential risk from soy isoflavones in soy protein isolate without adequate warning and information."

Soy is particularly problematic for infants, and soy infant formulas should be avoided. According to Dr. Daniel, soy formula contains phytoestrogens that can disrupt the baby's thyroid, reproductive development and toxic levels of manganese that can cause neurological and brain damage associated with ADD/ADHD and violent tendencies. Babies on soy formula are also at higher risk for gastrointestinal damage, allergies, asthma, poor mineral absorption and lower intelligence. It has been estimated that infants who are fed soy formula exclusively receive five birth control pills worth of estrogen every day! Most people think they are getting a healthy formula when they choose soy; indeed, if it is a formula for something, it most likely is a formula for their undoing.

So, question remains – what is the difference between soy in most products and the soy that gives rise to nattokinase. Well, in this regard, it is important to differentiate the difference between the health effects of fermented vs. non-fermented soy. Non-fermented soy products contain a chemical called *phytic acid*, which actually tends to block your ability to synthesize and nutrients. *Phytic acid* binds with certain nutrients, including iron, to inhibit their absorption. When soybeans are fermented into products like natto or tempeh, this effect of *phytic acid* is demonstrably reduced. The fermentation also creates probiotics – the "good" bacteria your body is absolutely dependent on, such as lactobacilli, which increase the quantity, availability, digestibility and assimilation of nutrients in your body. Interestingly, the fermentation process actually removes virtually all of the negative side effects of soy and converts it into a powerful health food.

In sum, there are actually some very good qualities to soy; however, these are found primarily in fermented soy products like tempeh, miso and natto and soybean sprouts. If you want to get some health benefits from soy, stick to these four and eliminate the processed soy milks, burgers, ice cream, cheese, and the multitude of other soy junk foods that are so readily masked as health foods.

A Final Word on Nattokinase

Dr. Martin Milner of the Center for Natural Medicine in Portland, Oregon and Dr. Kouhei Makise of the Imadeqawa Makise Clinica in Kyoto, Japan were able to launch a joint research project on nattokinase and write an extensive paper on their findings. "In all my years of research as a professor of cardiovascular and pulmonary medicine, natto and nattokinase represents the most exciting new development in the prevention and treatment of cardiovascular related diseases," Dr. Milner said. "We have finally found a potent natural agent that can thin and dissolve clots effectively, with relative safety and without side effects."

In short, with the discovery of nattokinase, you now have a safe, natural and very effective remedy for the prevention and management of heart problems which could very well spare you from hardened arteries, heart attack, stroke, angina, dementia and senility. In terms of heartbeat irregularities, your traditionally trained medical doctor has, will or would have told you to take aspirin to combat the risk of blood clots in the event you happen to have an attack of AFIB. Now, with nattokinase, you will achieve the benefits of the "aspirin strategy" but without the pitfalls.

STRATEGY #5 – WALK YOUR WAY OUT OF PALPITATIONS

This is an interesting strategy. Walking is a good, slow rhythmic movement exercise. Your body is designed to walk for long distances and for long periods at a time. People in other countries, such as Europe walk 10 to 50 times more than the average American. Walking (particularly outside on a nice sunny day) is probably one of the healthiest things you can do. Your lymphatic system is eliminating your toxins, your muscles are getting revitalized, and your body is flowing smoothly and rhythmically.

Walking is an amazing and quite effective strategy to signficantly reduce and usually eliminate the current onslaught of PCs and prevent them from occurring in the first place. Notice we said PCs, not AFIB. If you are having a lone AFIB experience, the situation is more serious and you should relax, as your heart rate will typically be too high and exercise will only make the situation worse. However, walking as a preventative measure, where you have a history of AFIB, is a good practice. Regularly walk at least 2 miles per day, and at least 4 to 5 times per week.

When you are having PCs, walking at a regular pace tends to change up the current state of the heart's rate and irregular beat. Walking steps up the heart rate, just a bit (as compared with anerobic exercise, such as weight lifting) and the consistent repetitive walking motion at a relatively slow pace frequently brings it into a normal sinus rhythm without palpitations. Many people have reported a sort of normalcy to the heart rhythm after walking a couple of miles.

Stress is a very frequent cause of irregular heartbeats. As I will discuss below, under "Strategy #7 – Miscellaneous Lifestyle Changes" involving the concept of stress, when you are under stressful situation, your parasympathetic nervous system frequently places you in the "fight or flight" syndrome you sometimes hear about. At the same time your body is such that your adrenal glands release adrenaline to allow you to "fight" in connection with a stressful situation.

The adrenaline is released through your body and, specifically though your heart muscle. However, while the adrenaline is supposed to provide you with a greater degree of oxygen to your cells, the chemical also has the side effect of getting in the way of the electrical conduction system of your heart cells.

Your heart cells generally give off an electical impulse independent of the natural pacemaker in your heart. Under normal circumstances, these "minor" impulses are usually overwhemed by the much stronger electrical charge of the natural pacemaker. But, when excessive adrenaline is pumped into the heart muscle, it can give enough extra "power" to the other cells so that when these minor charges are released, they are a lot stronger than what would otherwise be the case. The result is an interference with the natural pacemaker. This can cause heartbeat irregularties.

Your adrenal glands have not been taught by you to distinguish between physical fighting and mental stress and anguish. In most situations, it may not be practical or prudent to take "flight" or simply leave the stressful environment; however, when you do have an opportunity, it is submitted that walking in a relaxing manner away from the point of the stress simulates "flight", so that your body can regulate the release of adrenaline. Just as your body is tricked into going into a "fight or flight" condition, it can be tricked into receding from that state – through something as simple as walking. And, again, best of all, it's free.

However, walking will not always work, and you must be careful to distinguish what may be normal PCs and something more serious. Usually, what I try to do is walk slowly at an even pace to determine what is going on. If the palpitations go away in a short while, I will step it up a bit. For those readers familiar with walking speeds, I would start out at about 2.8 miles per hour, and maybe work up to 3.8 miles per hour. So, as a general rule, the more problemmatical the perceived PCs are, the slower you should walk. If they are very occasional and intermittent, then you could step it up a notch.

There is one very nice thing about this particular strategy – it's free!

STRATEGY #6 – INCREASE YOUR INTAKE OF WATER

When dealing with stress and the stressful experience of heart issues, it's important to take care of yourself physically as well as mentally. If your body is not well maintained, you will have fewer defenses to the ill effects of stress. One deficiency we commonly experience in times of stress is a lack of water. Your body is mostly water, and so this ongoing intake of water is essential to your every function. In his book *Your Body's Many Cries for Water*, F. Batmanghelidj notes that consuming adequate amounts of water is the only way of making sure that important hormones, chemical messengers and nutrients effectively reach your vital organs."

Stress, alcohol and caffeine all affect the amount of water and the speed in which your body loses water. Any of these factors, alone or in combination, could cause a small but critical shrinkage of your brain. This small shrinkage will impair neuromuscular coordination, decrease concentration, and slow thinking. Unfortunately, increased consumption of caffeine or alcohol is common in times of stress, resulting in a loss of water. Batmanghelidj notes that tea, coffee, alcohol, and manufactured beverages recognizably contain water, but in reality they are actually dehydrating agents because of their strong diuretic action on your kidneys. Such beverages get rid of the water they are dissolved in as well as more water from the reserves of your body. He further states that the "constant substituting of caffeine-containing drinks for water will deprive the body of its full capacity for the formation of hydroelectric energy…Excess caffeine intake will eventually exhaust the heart muscle because of its over-stimulation."

The lack of adequate water is an indicator of unknown disease conditions within your body. Unfortunately, medical practitioners have been taught to silence or mask these signals with chemical products, notably drugs.

When your body becomes dehydrated, it goes through a certain mobilization pattern of change. Notably, your body will try to seek out your natural water reserves. In so doing, this causes stress, which may necessarily cause further dehydration. The result is that your body begins to change by certain hormones being secreted. These hormones, particularly one called *vasopressin*, causes your capillaries to constrict and your blood pressure to rise as sort of a by-product of its otherwise normal job of filtering water into your cells. A chain reaction occurs and there becomes an increased risk that irregular heartbeats will result. The bottom line – dehydration is the number one stressor of the human body – or any living matter (F. Batmanghelidj).

Shockingly, if you are the average person, you drink only one cup of water each day. The rest of the water your body needs must be extracted from other liquids or foods you eat.

Small changes in the amount of water in your body can make a big difference. The average amount of water lost per day includes two cups through breathing, two cups through invisible perspiration, and six cups through elimination. More water could also be lost through exercise or hard work, excessively dry air, and alcohol and caffeine consumption.

I am sure you have heard, from many different sources that you are supposed to drink 8 cups (each cup being 8 ounces) of water per day. While it is true that there are many theories concerning how much water you need to consume each day to maintain good health, the misconception is that everyone needs to drink the same amount of water. But, everyone's size and metabolic makeup is different. Some people need more water than others. For example, if you weigh less (150 pounds or less), drink five cups per day. For every 20 pounds of body weight over 150, drink one additional cup. If you weigh over 250 pounds, drink as many as 2-13 cups.[22]

Things get a bit more complicated in what type of water to drink. Bottled spring water and filtered water are both good options. Also keep in mind that the spring (not "drinking") water should be bottled in clear polyethylene or glass containers, not the one-gallon plastic (PVC) containers that transfer far too many chemicals into the water. Filtered water can be obtained through low-cost filters.

Do not drink tap water or distilled water – period. Tap water should be avoided because it contains chlorine and may contain fluoride, as well as toxic substances that, with ongoing consumption, can have calamitous consequences for your body.

Some Very Good Reasons Not To Drink Tap Water

Arsenic is a well-known poison that has been the subject of murders for decades. After all, it is tasteless, colorless and odorless. A one-time oral dose of 60,000 ppb of arsenic will kill you. That's no more than 1/50 the weight of a penny, which shows how dangerous arsenic really is; however, it is unlikely you will get that much at one time. The sad truth is that arsenic can kill you slowly without you being the subject of any murder. Typically, it will be absorbed into your body over many, many years, through drinking water and through food and the air you breathe.

The scary thing is that arsenic occurs naturally in some soil and rock. When water comes in contact with arsenic in soil or rocks, it's absorbed naturally. Industrial processes such as mining, smelting and coal-fired electric power plants contribute to the presence of arsenic in your water. Arsenic can either be discharged directly into rivers and streams or pumped into the air. When arsenic is pumped into the air, it travels with the wind before settling back into lakes and rivers. Or, if arsenic settles on the ground, it's carried into the underground water supply by rain or melting snow.

Arsenic is also used in agricultural pesticides and chemicals used to preserve wood. The residue from this process can be drained into rivers, lakes and underground water supplies.

According to the World Health Organization, arsenic is very common in ground water across the United States. The possible health effects of consuming even low levels of arsenic are skin cancer, nervous system damage, diabetes, circulatory diseases, high blood pressure, and reduced intelligence in children. And, if that wasn't enough, studies have also linked long-term arsenic exposure to an increased risk of cancer of the bladder, lungs, liver and other organs. Arsenic can also damage your chromosomes, which house the genetic material inside the cells of your body.

It's believed the side effects from arsenic exposure in drinking water typically take years to develop. Much of it depends on the concentration of arsenic to which you are exposed. Most arsenic leaves your body within three days of exposure. But the arsenic that remains is stored in the brain, bones and tissue and continues to do serious damage. The only good news is that arsenic is not well absorbed through the skin.

Have you ever heard of the metal barium? Well, barium is just as dangerous to your health as those other metals and shows up regularly in public water supplies. Because barium is used often in so many manufacturing operations (paint, tile, rubber, soap, linoleum, spark plugs, fireworks, cosmetics and a host of others including rat poison), a lot of waste is produced that needs to be removed from the environment. In 2002, the Environmental Protection Agency reported more than 222 million pounds of barium and barium compounds were legally released into the air, wells, lakes, rivers and landfills. Ten states account for about half of all legal barium released in this country with Texas leading the way with 17.1 million pounds.

Exposure to small amounts of barium, dissolved in water, may cause a person to experience breathing difficulties, increased blood pressure, heart rhythm changes, and other heart damage, not to mention stomach irritation, muscle weakness, alterations in nerve reflexes and damage to your brain, liver, and kidney.

In short, stay as far away from tap water as you can, unless it is otherwise absolutely necessary.

Distilled water should also be avoided. Distillation is the process in which water is boiled, evaporated and the vapor condensed. On the positive side, distilled water is free of dissolved minerals and, because of this, has the special property of being able to actively absorb toxic substances from the body and eliminate them. In fact, studies validate the benefits of drinking distilled water when one is seeking to cleanse or detoxify the system for short periods of time (a few weeks at a time). However, fasting using distilled water can be dangerous because of the rapid loss of electrolytes (sodium, potassium, chloride) and trace minerals like magnesium, deficiencies of which can cause heart beat irregularities and high blood pressure. Cooking foods in distilled water pulls the minerals out of them and lowers their nutrient value. Moreover, distilled water is an active absorber and when it comes into contact with air, it absorbs carbon dioxide, making it acidic. The more distilled water a person drinks, the higher the body acidity becomes. According to the U.S. Environmental Protection Agency, "distilled water, being essentially mineral-free, is very aggressive, in that it tends to dissolve substances with which it is in contact. Notably, carbon dioxide from the air is rapidly absorbed, making the water acidic and even more aggressive. Many metals are dissolved by distilled water."

The most toxic commercial beverages that people consume (i.e. cola beverages and other soft drinks) are made from distilled water. Because it has the wrong, suffice it to say, chemical structure (meaning ionization, pH, polarization and oxidation potential), and can drain your body of necessary minerals. It has been linked to hair loss, which is often associated with certain mineral deficiencies.

The most toxic commercial beverages that people consume (i.e. cola beverages and other soft drinks in bottles and cans) are made from distilled water. Studies have consistently shown that heavy consumers of soft drinks (with or without sugar) spill huge amounts of calcium, magnesium and other trace minerals into the urine. The more mineral loss, the greater the risk for coronary artery disease, high blood pressure and a long list of degenerative diseases generally associated with premature aging.[23]

Finally, drink water at room temperature if possible, as ice-cold water can harm the delicate lining of your stomach. Drink the appropriate amounts of water, and everything is much more likely to function at optimal levels, including your heart. If you do not drink enough water, and over the short term you will experience routine fatigue, dry skin, headaches and constipation; over the longer term, every body function will degrade more quickly. It really is as simple as that.

Now, in terms of heart irregularities, you should increase your intake of water when you have an attack of palpitations or even AFIB. You will be amazed that there is a direct correlation between triggering heartbeat irregularities and your intake of water. If you are like most people, you are dehydrated. This means that your cells do not have enough fluid. This can actually affect your energy levels and the quality of your sleep, but the major impact on your body is that water flushes the toxins and waste material out of your body and out of your cells.

You see, a living cell can last a very long time (much longer than you can ever imagine) if you just keep them cleaned and properly nourished. When a cell is properly maintained in this fashion, it excretes wastes and toxins, and really does not show the signs of aging. That is why water is so important to your heart health. I have found that this "flushing" of your bodily liquids eliminates the toxins and the allergens that may be causing the irregular heartbeats.

Also, when you increase your intake of water, obviously you will have a desire to urinate more frequently. I have also determined that consuming enough water to produce at least three urinations will frequently provide positive results in terms of lessening or eliminating any onslaught of irregular heartbeats. This also probably has to do with the changes in blood pressure in connection with your kidney filtration and urination process. Interestingly, this is partially caused by a certain regulation mechanism associated with your kidneys, called your *renin-angiotensin system* ("RA system"), which I will more particularly describe in Chapter 10).

In fact, when you lack enough water, your RA system becomes quite active. When you get enough water its activity is decreased. Until that time, your RA system causes the tightening of your capillaries and your vascular system as a whole. Your kidneys have a sense of recognizing the degree of fluid flow and the filtration pressure to make urine. If this filtration pressure is not adequate for urine filtration and release, the RA system will tighten your blood vessels at the site of your kidneys and influence all parts of your body. This whole process readily and easily leads to hypertension, which can further lead to palpitations and irregular heartbeats of all sorts.[24]

So, how do you know if you are getting enough water? Well, Batmanghelidj points out that the normal color of your urine should not be dark. Instead, it should be colorless to light yellow. If it becomes dark yellow or even orange, you are probably dehydrated. This means that your kidneys are working very hard to get rid of your toxins.

STRATEGY # 7 – MISCELLANEOUS LIFESTYLE CHANGES

Get More and Better Exercise

Include exercise in your daily routine. Regular exercise not only lowers the resting heart rate, but it also burns adrenaline, a hormone that causes an increase in heart rate. However, if you are predisposed to arrhythmias and palpitations, you need to be careful with respect to your exercise routine. Generally, aerobics are an excellent form of rhythmic exercise for your body and heart in particular. Sprinting type exercise, like tennis and racket sports can be a bit problematical. The "spurting" nature of these activities tends to trigger adrenaline more inconsistently, which sometimes takes the heart muscle by surprise and causes palpitations. This can be not only annoying and psychologically disturbing, it can also potentially trigger AFIB. Regarding weight training, which is more of an anaerobic exercise, you should undertake extreme care. Lifting heavy weights places a tremendous strain on your heart and could trigger irregular heartbeats. These beats could evolve into AFIB. This is good reason for you to engage in judicious strength training. Notably, do push-ups, pull-ups, and sit-ups with minimal or no weight. Try isometrics. However, if you have to lift weights, lift light weights and increase your reps.

Stop Inhaling Burning Tobacco Leaves Laced with Highly Toxic Chemicals

Yes, that's the long way of saying STOP SMOKING, which has turned into an overused cliché. Nicotine is a stimulant that can cause heart rate to soar, so it is exceedingly beneficial to quit smoking. In the past, smoking was thought of as increasing the risk for lung cancer. However, modern medicine has clearly identified smoking as a major culprit in increasing the risks of heart disease and heart related conditions. More than 400,000 Americans die each year of smoking-related illnesses, and many of these deaths can be traced back to the effect that smoking has had on the heart and blood vessels. Smoking increases your heart rate and the chance of irregular beats, and tightens major arteries. All of this makes your heart work harder. Smoking also raises your blood pressure, which increases the risk of stroke if you already have heart problems.

While quitting smoking, recognizably, is no easy task, there is one relatively simplistic thought process that you might employ to give you a different perspective on your cigarette smoking habit. Take a good, long and hard look at the cigarette you are smoking and imagine it being symbolic of one of your body parts, like your lungs or your heart. Look at the cigarette and observe how it is burning and how this material (consisting of dead plant life, notably trees and leaves that were once living matter), is now on fire and being burned to a crisp. Then, think of how the same thing is happening in your body – you are burning it up (actually, a long slow burn) and literally causing your life to go up in smoke!

Get More Quality Sleep

With proper rest, your cells are allowed the opportunity to recharge and rejuvenate. You eliminate your toxins and you heal while you sleep.

Sleep is as important as food, water and air. Quantity and quality are very important. Most people need between 7.5 to 8.5 hours of uninterrupted sleep. If you are either getting up too early or wanting to press the snooze alarm in the morning, you are not getting the sleep you need. This could be due to not enough time in bed, external disturbances, or a sleep disorder. While you sleep, your body secretes hormones that affect your mood, energy, memory, and concentration. Recent research suggests that if sleep deprivation is long-term – whether because of lifestyle choices or sleep disorders – it may increase the severity of age-related chronic disorders such as diabetes and high blood pressure, not to mention irregular heartbeats. Whatever the reason for sleep loss, research has shown that it takes a toll on you both mentally and physically.

One of the most profound ways to reduce the impact of arrhythmias is to get better sleep. Sounds simple to say, but it is becoming tougher and tougher to accomplish. You are not alone if you are one of the millions of Americans not getting your 8 hours of sleep per night.

What to Avoid

There are some lifestyle changes you can make to get better, longer more qualitative sleep. To begin with avoid alcoholic beverages in the late evening, particularly near bedtime. Alcohol tends to make you sleepy, but it's also metabolized quickly – within two to three hours for moderate doses. So you'll have a rebound effect. You may sleep soundly for the first couple of hours but then toss and turn later. Alcohol can cause quite a bit of restlessness during the night.

If you are like many people, you drink coffee after having a few drinks to get you alert. However, caffeine and nicotine have substances in them that will keep you awake. Also, while exercise will be great for better sleep, do not exercise near (usually within 3 hours of) your bedtime.

Avoid liquids before bed, as it will interfere with your sleep and it will tend to wake you up from your bladder being full and desirous of emptying. Moreover, large meals in the two hours before bedtime could cause indigestion. And, above all, don't take a nap early in the evening since it will disrupt your sleeping pattern for the night. Naps can be good, but the American Academy of Sleep Medicine recommends napping before 3 p.m. and for no longer than an hour so that it doesn't interfere with falling asleep at night.

Another trick involves the supplements your may be taking, other than the supplements referred to in this Chapter 5. This may include multi-vitamins, hormones like DHEA, and cognitive enhancement supplements amongst others. These agents tend to keep you up at night and they should be taken early in the day (before 2 p.m.) if at all possible. If you take anything later in the day, restrict it to your mineral supplements like magnesium and others. As for liquids, try to restrict your water intake past 7 p.m. at night, since this will lessen the chance of waking up in the middle of the night having to go to the bathroom.

Avoid watching TV, working on your laptop, or reading in bed because you want to condition yourself to understand that your bedroom is a place to sleep, not a recreational center. Also, try to avoid sleep interruptions by not sleeping with your pets, closing your door, and minimizing light and noise. Finally, in terms of what to do and not to do before bed, check you medications, particularly those that treat colds and allergies, heart disease, high blood pressure, and pain, as they might be keeping you awake. Also, avoid bright light around the house before bed. Using dimmer switches in living rooms and bathrooms before bed can be helpful (dimmer switches can be set to maximum brightness for morning routines).

Routines

Bedtime routines are helpful for good sleep. If you can't get to sleep for over 30 minutes, get out of bed and do something boring in dim light till you are sleepy. Keep routines on your normal schedule. A cup of herbal tea (chamomile is a good relaxing one that I use frequently) an hour before bed can be part of a nice routine. Avoid looking at the clock if you wake up in the middle of the night. Seeing the time of day (particularly at that early hour) can cause anxiety. This is very difficult for most of us, so turn the clock away from your eyes so you would have to turn it to see the time. You may decide not to make the effort and go right back to sleep. Keep your bedroom at a comfortable temperature. Not too warm and not too cold. Cooler is better than warmer. If you have problems with noise in your environment you can use a white noise generator. An old fan, or better yet, a noisy air purifier, would work fine. Absent those items, there are plenty of companies who make noise simulation products.

Getting bright light, typically from the sun, when you get up will also help. Interestingly, bright light in the morning at a regular time should help you feel sleepy at the same time every night.

Now, in terms of your palpitations, temporary insomnia is a factor that might enter into the equation of significantly interfering with your sleep. Temporary insomnia can be caused by noise or a stressful event like bad news at work, the loss of a job, or a death in the family. We will talk more about stress in a few more pages. But, if you have trouble getting these interferences out of your mind when you go to sleep, try some self-hypnosis stress relieving audio tapes/CDs right before bed. Also, getting more oxygen during sleep should help your sleeping. Try using one of the various brands of breathing strips that you place over your nose (it's the kind that you see many of the pro football players use to increase the flow of air through their nasal passages).

If you cannot get enough quality sleep, particularly at first, it is also important to get enough rest. Rest is the next best thing to sleep. If you are like most people you do not get enough rest during the day. You get up, work all day, come home, go to bed late and never get a good, full eight hours of restful sleep. This results in your body never having a chance to heal and recharge. Take a laptop computer and leave it on until the battery died and then recharged it the next time. Then take another laptop and always put it on standby or "sleep" mode, when you are not using it. You will learn that the battery life will probably be much longer by not keeping it on all the time. Your body is much like a battery-powered device, needs rest. Get enough rest and sleep and you will have much more energy and the degree to which you get ill would be reduced significantly.

Sleep Apnea

Sleep apnea is characterized by a number of involuntary breathing pauses during a single night's sleep. It may be as many as 20 to 30 or more events per hour involving breathing lapses between 10 seconds to one minute. During the sleep apnea event, you are unable to breathe in oxygen and to exhale carbon dioxide, resulting in low levels of oxygen and increased levels of carbon dioxide in your blood. The reduction in your oxygen levels and increase in your carbon dioxide alert your brain to resume breathing and cause you to become aroused. With each arousal, a signal is sent from your brain to your upper airway muscles to open the airway. Your breathing is then resumed, often with a loud snort or gasp or choking sensation. In other words, these events are almost always accompanied by snoring (keep in mind that if you snore, it does not mean you have sleep apnea; conversely, if you do not snore, most likely you do not have sleep apnea).

The frequent interruptions of deep, restorative sleep often lead to early morning headaches and excessive daytime sleepiness. The frequent arousals, although necessary for your breathing to restart, prevent you from getting enough restorative, deep sleep and may be one of the sources of your irregular heartbeats.

It is estimated that as many as 18 million Americans have sleep apnea. It is more common in men, although it may be under-diagnosed in women. The risk of recurrent AFIB is doubled in people with untreated sleep apnea, according to a Mayo Clinic study in 2005 as reported in the medical journal *Circulation*. In the study, obstructive sleep apnea, in which there is a blockage of the airway, was the single factor most closely associated with recurrence of AFIB.

Prescription Drugs

Prescription drugs for sleep (often called "hypnotic drugs") act in areas of the brain to help promote sleep. There have been advances with the development of more short-acting drugs to decrease drowsy spillover effects in the morning. *Sonata (zaleplon)*, for example, is a drug designed to help you fall asleep faster, but not for keeping you asleep. *Ambien (zolpidem)* is an example of a drug indicated for both getting to sleep and staying asleep. In my particular case, I have found these drugs do not work that well. Moreover, hypnotic drugs are potentially addictive. Generally, their use is limited to 10 days or less, and the longest that they are approved for use is about 30 days. Having stated that, there are some new drugs now being marketed like *Lunesta (eszopiclone)* that are approved for longer use. But, the fact remains, like most drugs, hypnotic drugs are "band-aid cures" for serious behavioral, physiological and/or psychological problems that cry out for more substantive long-term solutions. They might be all right at best in an isolated temporary situation; however, they should not be relied upon as a medium or long-term solution.

Get More Natural Sunlight

If there were anything that would be the 8th strategy, in and of itself, it would have to be sunlight in terms of heart health and even controlling irregular heartbeats. Yes, believe it or not, I submit that exposure to sunlight is an inexpensive lifestyle change that can affect the quality and quantity of your palpitations. Much of this notion is based upon studies that have shown that natural sunlight can actually significantly lower your blood pressure due to certain hormones being released from the proper synthesis of vitamin D. By regulating the level of calcium in your blood, vitamin D influences your nervous system in a positive way, by causing calcium to aid your nerve impulse transmission and your muscle contraction. This has a positive effect on the regulation of the normal sinus rhythm of your heart. (see also Chapter 10, "Taking the Pressure Off Your Blood").

Interestingly, author Richard Hobday, in his book called *The Healing Sun* states that "not only does sunlight lower blood pressure and cholesterol levels, but the results of tests....show that exposure to ultraviolet radiation can also increase the amount of blood ejected from the heart [remember, we called that *cardiac output*] by 39%." He further points out that more people die of heart attacks in the winter months than the rest of the year and deaths from heart disease become more common the farther you live from the equator.

Yes, getting more sunlight is yet another significant bit of information that clearly goes against the grain of the recommendations you have received in the past to avoid any sun exposure, particularly by the mainstream dermatological community. On the contrary, you, and every one else, need sunlight to stay healthy.

The advice of the traditional medical community to stay out of the sun, because the sun will cause cancer, may actually be one of the major reasons why there actually is actually an <u>increase</u> in heart disease! You and everyone else needs sunlight and when you don't receive it your health may decline.

And, on the issue of sunscreens, Hobday contends that they really give people a false sense of security because most of them block out essentially the UVB rays, which were thought to be the most dangerous. However, more and more studies have shown that the UVA rays, which were once thought to be safe, actually penetrate much deeper into the skin and cause collagen and elastin damage and cause wrinkles to appear, not to mention leading to the development of premature aging. UVA rays are also known to be linked to malignant melanoma. Sunscreens, according to Hobday, are designed to protect against sunburn, but there is no scientific proof that sunscreens are designed to protect against basal cell carcinoma or malignant melanoma (in fact, he contends that basal cell and its cousin, squamous cell carcinoma, are the result of repeated exposures to the sun when your body isn't ready to handle **excessive** sun exposure).

According to a heavily annotated report in Life Extension Magazine in June of 2005, *Why Sunscreens Do Not Fully Prevent Skin Cancer* (D. Keifer), recent studies suggest that sunscreen use may not reduce the risk of melanoma because they have little impact on reducing the free radicals generated in response to solar radiation exposure the deadliest of skin cancers. "In other words, while sunburn-inducing ultraviolet-B [UVB] rays can be blocked, other kinds of solar radiation continue to inflict DNA damage that can result in skin cancer. These same free radicals also contribute to skin aging." (D. Keifer)

Moreover, some health authorities have very recently suggested (in 2005) that the rigorous use of sunscreen may paradoxically result in a vitamin D deficiency – the vitamin you are actually trying to gain by being in the sun in the first place.

So, you are grossly mistaken that you can safely sit or play in the sun as long as you are covered with a commercial sunscreen. Heck, this little tip may worth the price of this book alone!

Hobday contends that the current problems with sunlight, skin cancer and premature aging is more to do with the environmental factors (pollution, alcohol consumption, cigarette smoke, just to name a few) and the highly refined diet of most Americans – a diet that promotes considerable free radical activity (which you will read more about below in Part II). For now, suffice it to say that free radicals are highly reactive molecular fragments that can be very destructive when combined with molecules in your body. The sunlight burning the free radicals is what causes the problems (cancer, heart disease, arthritis, etc.) – not the sun itself. And, the less free radical activity you have in your body, the better. Without stealing too much of the thunder of Chapter 8-10 below, consuming substantial amounts of antioxidants, such as vitamin A, B, C, and E, together with selenium, bioflavonoids, beta-carotene, zinc, and a bunch of other compounds, are highly useful in preventing free radical activity or protecting your body once the free radicals have formed.

Just use common sense guidelines when in the sun and always avoid getting sun burned. You should probably limit exposure during the peak hours of the day. There are other rules that Hobday recommends. He notes that you (i) should not cram all your sun exposure into a short period (rather, plan longer term), (ii) don't sunbathe in very hot temperature, (iii) don't cover yourself with sunscreen or sunblock unless you will be outside for a prolonged period of time (and even then, just use a good sunblock or natural, antioxidant-laden sunscreen or clothing), (iv) wear a hat, and (v) pay close attention to the way your skin tans or burns and adjust accordingly. On the matter of sunscreen, I would be remiss to suggest a particular one formulated by the Life Extension Foundation called

Total Sun Protection Cream, which is loaded with topical antioxidants and powerful sunray-blocking agents.

Thus, against that background, it is submitted that a short exposure, like 30-45 minutes a day, to sunshine goes a long way in preventing palpitations. And, even better, use that 30-45 minutes a day to walk in the sunshine. And, above all, it's free!

Reduce Your Stress and Anxiety Levels

Stress and anxiety can trigger a myriad of problems in your body that are typically caused by a myriad of problems in your life. The concept of stress isn't new to anyone. But few people truly know what stress is. Physical stress is the depletion of the body's resources by illness or exhaustion. The most devastating stress, however, is psychological and emotional stress. There are many sources of emotional stress: family problems, social obligations, life changes, work, decision-making, and phobias.

Emotional stress is powerful and debilitating because it takes away any sense of control you have over your life. And, this feeling of control over your environment and yourself is one of your most basic human needs. If it isn't met, emotional or physical illness can result. A number of studies directly link stress and heart disease. Stress can cause a lack of blood flow to your heart and increase your risk of death if you already have coronary heart disease. This is because when you are under stress, your heart goes faster and your blood pressure rises, increasing your demand for oxygen. When your heart is diseased, it cannot pump blood fast enough to supply the oxygen that you need, and, unfortunately, the result may be angina or chest pain. Also, your nervous system releases extra hormones (such as adrenaline). These hormones raise your blood pressure, which can injure the linings of your arteries. When your arteries heal, the walls may harden or thicken, making it easier for plaque to build up. Blood clots are more likely to form during times of stress and could block an artery already narrowed by plaque. This may lead to a heart attack.

Stress and anxiety can also cause palpitations and arrythmias. This is due to your adrenal glands releasing adrenaline because you are under such stress. It's that "fight or flight" syndrome you sometimes hear about. Your body is such that your adrenals release adrenaline to allow you to "fight" in connection with a stressful situation. Unfortunately, if you are like most people, your adrenal glands have not been taught by you to distinguish between physical fighting and mental stress and anguish. You know, it's when you get into a disagreement with your boss, when you are arguing vehemently with your spouse, when you get stark raving mad with inconsiderate, negligent drivers on the roadways, or when you are called to be a witness in a court hearing. It can also happen when you are lifting weights or playing sports of any variety. While you can, in some situations, take "flight" or simply leave the stressful environment, it may not be practical or prudent in many situations.

The adrenaline is released through your body and, specifically though your heart muscle. However, while the adrenaline is supposed to provide you with a greater degree of oxygen to your cells, the chemical also has the side effect of getting in the way of the electrical conduction system of your heart cells according to Dr. Philip J. Podrid, MD, Professor of Medicine, Boston University School of Medicine.

You see, your heart cells generally give off an electical impulse independent of the natural pacemaker in your heart. Under normal circumstances, these "minor" impulses are usually overwhemed by the much stronger electical charge of the natural pacemaker. But, when excessive adrenaline is pumped into the heart muscle, it can give enough extra "power" to the other cells so that when these minor charges are released, they are a lot stronger than what would otherwise be the case. The result is an interference with the natural pacemaker. This can cause heartbeat irregularties.

Reducing stress and anxiety can help lessen your heart palpitations. This can either be by undergoing stress reduction techniques before you find yourself in a stress or anxious situation, such as meditation, exercise, yoga, etc. However, that is easier said than done for most people. So, the goal is to reduce the stress and anxiety when you find yourself in an anxious moment.

Using Simple Breathing Techniques

Try breathing exercises or deep relaxation (a step-by-step process of tensing and then relaxing every muscle group in your body) at the time of your heartbeat sensations.

Another sure fire way is to simply take long slow deep breaths one after another. Inhale slowly and exhale slowly. It will usually take between 3 and 6 of these breaths to normalize you. If they persist, continue this procedure of deep breathing in sets of 3 to 6 deep, long breaths.

For a full scale attack on the problem, combine both of the above techniques. First, find a comfortable place to sit down. Second, take a long deep breath, but instead of exhaling, you hold your breath at the end of the long inhale for about 4 seconds. Then, you exhale slowly and count silently to about 7 or 8 counts, and think of the word "R E L A X" at each count down on the exhale. You will be amazed at how this relaxes you. Also, consider practicing yoga or tai chi on a regular basis to reduce the frequency of your palpitations. All of these strategies will tend to relax you and prevent adrenaline from being produced to cause irregular beats.

Utilize the Emotional Freedom Technique™ (EFT)

This a technique that was developed by Gary Craig. The Emotional Freedom Technique™ (EFT) centers around exploiting certain subtle energies of your body and how to reduce negative emotions, reduce pain and even address illnesses. Accordingly, EFT is like an emotional form of acupuncture except that you don't use needles. Instead, you tap certain parts of the upper part of your body with your fingertips (about 10-12 times) to stimulate certain meridian energy points while you are "tuned in" to your problem. In fact, on his website (www.emofree.com), Mr. Craig allows you to download considerable free information that will enable you to utilize much of what is needed for addressing the condition of stress and how it may necessarily affect heart arrhythmias. Mr. Craig touts that EFT addresses all types of ailments, but we are using it here for just a limited purpose.

There is actually a website that pictorially shows EFT (www.mercola.com/forms/eftcourse3.htm). Suffice it to say that the technique involves simple tapping of 3 or 4 of your fingertips on various places on your body – your forehead, the top of your head, the bone on the outside of your eye, the bone under your eye, the bone under your nose, your chin bone, near your mid breast bone, your sides (4 inches below the armpit, and your wrists. All in all, this sounds somewhat unconventional (to say the least), but it seems to work for me and it might just work for you.

Don't Let Stress Take Control – Talk It Out

The pressure for you to perform in today's world is intense. As a result, you may work long hours (whether it's on the job or at home as a homemaker) and take on much more than you can bear. You might juggle multiple roles throughout the day and sacrifice sleep or personal time just so you can get everything done. The stress of living in today's environment is greater than ever before. Whether it's driving a car, worrying about money, arguing with friends, spouses, or co-workers, watching gruesome movies, listening to or reading the news (which now seems to be about nothing but crimes), your stress levels are increased.

Correcting your attitude and taking control of your thoughts may be one of the best ways to control stress. Positive thoughts create a chemical reaction in your body that promotes healing and well-being. Negative thoughts create high levels of stress and promote chemical reactions leading to illness and disease. Interestingly, I have a relative who sadly got hooked early in life on cigarettes. He is now 60 years old and he has contracted emphysema and a host of other illnesses from urinary tract problems to prostate problems to high blood pressure and more. On top of all that, he takes 10–20 prescription drugs (pills) a day not including non-prescription drugs. By some accounts, he should not really be alive. However, with all that, he still works very hard and is productive at what he does. Remarkably, he has been able to be a very positive, optimistic person that doesn't take life that seriously. He is light-hearted and generous. He seems to greet each day with a spirit of thankfulness. His attitude seems to have really made the difference, as his thoughts and outlook on life have seemed to counteract his man-made health problems, and his thoughts have positively affected his health (or certainly counteracted many of the unhealthy things that he has done to his body).

Many times saying "no" to a particular demand on your life is difficult and this results in increased stress, both at work and at home. You are anxious to please others, so you put your own needs aside. You don't realize that no one can be on call 24 hours a day, and that we all need some personal time to rest and rejuvenate.

The next time someone demands more than you can give, remember that you have to take care of yourself first. You simply can't handle everything. Say "no" tactfully while respecting the other person and letting him or her know that you care. While you may feel some initial guilt for denying the request, that feeling will quickly pass and your stress level will remarkably be reduced.

Also, listening to your body will usually help you identify that you are under stress (like, of course, having arrhythmias or irregular heartbeats). When this happens, you must become responsible for your health and your stress. Relying on your doctor to help or provide a solution is the proverbial "cop out." The real solution lies with you and with your own awareness and responsibility for your health. This responsibility may involve doing some things that are difficult for you, such as changing your diet, stopping smoking, cease drinking coffee, cutting out alcohol, learning to control emotions, etc. Whatever change is necessary for you, your body will tell you. You need only to listen.

Allow your subconscious mind to communicate with your hormones and your heart to relieve stress and to otherwise calm down any irregular beats. First, you need to find a comfortable quiet place and incorporate some of the breathing techniques noted in the section immediately above. Listen to some soft, relaxing music or obtain some audio tapes/CDs that are designed to place your mind in a relaxed state of mind.

To reduce emotional stress, your heart needs respect, encouragement, appreciation and love. Again, while there are tapes/CDs designed to do this, you might incorporate the following affirmation to yourself:

> "I want my heart to help me be peaceful and to create an emotional barrier that protects me from everything that I may be fighting with. Within my heart there is an infinite intelligence that is responsive to my needs". [Now, raise an issue specifically that is causing you concerns and ask your heart to help you alleviate your fears, frustrations and annoyances. In other words, pose a question to your heart or discuss a problem that's causing you stress. Think back over the recent period of your strife or even over your life and identify the most painful experiences you have had – the ones you thought you needed to just get away from it all. What was that mistake or event? What message did the event trigger in your mind? Then, acknowledge the event, forgive yourself for it, and then release it and the accompanying stress from your heart.]

Your heart will reciprocate with the proper answer and/or action. By doing this, you are telling your creative part of your brain to allow you to find new solutions to your problems. The more you become aware of your heart and what it tells you to do, the less stress you will experience. You will achieve a sense of peace and calmness knowing that you are doing what is best for you. Then, relax for 10 to 15 more minutes and then go about your daily activities. You should be refreshed and revitalized.

Things to Stay Away From

Caffeine causes an increase in heart rate, even after just one cup of coffee or soda pop, so drink decaffeinated beverages and avoid other sources of caffeine. And, along these lines, reduce, and ideally eliminate, your use of, and reliance upon, processed sugars of all forms. Processed sugar is one the most dangerous substances known to man and can easily trigger releases of insulin and adrenaline, which in turn can upset the normal sinus rhythm in your heart. For more on the devastating effects of sugar, see "Chapter 8 – Lowering Your Cholesterol and Your Drugs Without Lowering Your Standards – Naturally."

Another thing to consider not having around you is mercury. Do you remember the discussion on toxic mercury under Strategy #1? Well, mercury vapors from amalgam "silver" fillings in your teeth are continually released in your mouth and increased when you chew food or gum. Studies have found people with these fillings can have mercury vapor concentrations 10 times higher than those in people without them. Also, simple activities such as chewing gum, drinking hot liquids and brushing teeth can further increase the release of mercury. You need to replace these "silver" amalgam fillings in your teeth.

Therefore, if you are in a position to do this, and want to do it the right way, where you won't get worse, contact a dentist who is particularly specialized in removing mercury-based fillings – one who undertakes special precautions to prevent further mercury from getting into your tissues during the removal process. This book is not intended to be a treatise on dentistry – holistic, biological or otherwise – but it would behoove you to do some research on these precautions. If your dentist does not appreciate mercury toxicity they will probably not implement special precautions, like room air to you by nasal cannula, rubber dams and high-pressure suction to suck out the mercury vapors that are released by drilling.

Although just about any dentist is technically qualified to replace your amalgam fillings, only a small percentage have the protocol in place to properly reduce your risk of mercury exposure during the removal process.

WHAT I WOULD DO

So, in light of the above, what would I do if I wanted to prevent, reduce the symptoms of, or eliminate irregular heartbeats? Well, in the form of a summary, let's divide the subject into two sections – prevention and addressing the dealing with benign arrhythmias. Again, this is not medical advice. This is my own opinion based upon the information researched, numerous studies reviewed and my own personal experiences.

Prevention

Take fish oil (containing mercury-free omega-3 fatty acids) and CoQ10 religiously. I take, for preventative measures 1400 mg. of EPA, 1000 mg. of DHA, 200 mg. of other fatty acids daily. This mixture also contains sesame seed extract, which has shown to enhance the absorption and benefits of the fish oil.

Also, get plenty of magnesium or as much as is tolerable (500-1500 mg. daily). For preventative measures, I would consume about 1400 to 2000 mg of nattokinase daily. I would try to drink as much non-tap, non-distilled water as you can when taking these and other supplements that is part of your daily regimen. In addition to that, I would try very hard to consume at least the water quantities noted above under Strategy #6. And, above all, I would take daily walks, especially in natural sunlight (over a short period of time, like 30-45 minutes). And, if I had to create the ultimate "health trip", while walking listen to relaxing music (whether or not in natural sunlight) or a subliminal tape on relaxation and stress reduction.

I would exercise wisely without the use of heavy weight lifting and vary exercises as much as possible. Sleeping better is probably one of the best things that can be done to prevent PCs and AFIB. I would focus on sleeping better by incorporating many of the sleep suggestions noted above. And, I would be aware of problems that will infringe on natural sleeping patterns, such as sleep apnea. I would use breathing and other relaxation techniques to relieve stress, which should also cause better sleep.

Surprisingly, many of the suggestions noted above are actually free, that is, it won't cost you anything – like breathing, sleeping, exercising, getting more natural sunlight and, to a limited degree, drinking water with fairly inexpensive water filters. Big business cannot make money on these things so their benefits are significantly downplayed and have been for quite some time. In fact, avoiding smoking and caffeine will even save you quite a bit of money. Magnesium and fish oil can be bought thriftily, while nattokinase and Co Q10 are typically a bit more expensive.

In other words, overall, the seven natural and safe ways are fairly inexpensive to implement in your life.

Addressing the Symptoms

When one or more palpitations occur it is important to recognize what they are in the first place. As noted above, a medical doctor (typically a cardiologist) is well suited to diagnose the problem and determine if the irregular beats are benign or the result of some other, more serious heart ailment. If you have not had a medical doctor determine the nature of your irregular beats, then it is wise to consult with such a professional. If you have already done that, and are familiar with the nature and classification of your beats, then this is what I would do, assuming that you know that you are having PCs or the beginnings of an attack of AFIB.

First, try to determine the type of irregular beat. In most cases it should be PVCs. Second, sit down in a comfortable chair and try to relax. Take your blood pressure with a good quality blood pressure machine and compare it with what is normal for you.

Third, I would take one or two fish oil pills along with a magnesium pill, especially if I have not completed my daily regimen of those supplements. Even still, another one should not hurt me. I would also take a B-complex pill and one or two pills of a herbal formulation that I have not mentioned yet, notably Herbal Cardiovascular Formula. It contains bromelain, curcumin, ginger and a couple of other ingredients. I discuss it more in detail in the next section, *My Personal Regimen and Success Story*. Along with all that, I would start drinking bottled or filtered water (at least 3 glasses).

Fourth, I would try the breathing exercises noted above, in an attempt to get in as much oxygen as possible.

Fifth, I would try using the EFT tapping techniques to instantly relieve stress. If that still does not calm me down, I would try walking slowly at a moderate even pace. If the palpitations do not occur when I am walking (one or two palpitations may still be all right) then I should be able to walk myself out of the problem, along with the other measures discussed above. If the palpitations continue to occur while walking, I will stop, sit back down and try to relax – breathing long and slow, drinking water, Sometimes it takes between 30 minutes and as long as 8 hours for the symptoms to go away. However, using the above techniques should greatly shorten that process.

If the palpitations are frequent, irregular and continual, it may be an AFIB attack. The best way that I have found to handle that is to try and relax as much as possible, drink water, urinate as much as possible and wait out the storm (typically a 1-9 hour waiting period before your heart normalizes). AFIB is one type of benign arrhythmia (assuming it is benign) that is typically cured by the passage of time.

Now, the traditional mainstream medical community does have a treatment for benign AFIB when it happens, but it involves a couple of drugs, one of which is Tambacor (*flecainide*), the drug that had some very real dangerous side effects. In very healthy people, it has shown to shorten the period of AFIB, but it is wise to consult your cardiologist about the use of this drug in your particular case.

The best approach, of course, is to simply keep AFIB from happening in the first place by employing the techniques discussed in Strategies #1–7 discussed above.

MY PERSONAL REGIMEN AND SUCCESS STORY

In General

Now that I have outlined many of the techniques to avoid and alleviate irregular heartbeats, the question you might ask is how has this helped me. Well, it has helped me a lot. My palpitations are controlled, my blood pressure is excellent, and demonstrably down from what it was prior to the time when I began this regimen (from about 135/82 to about 115/73), my cholesterol is at very good levels, and other key markers such as homocysteine and C-reactive protein are all at perfect levels. While I was never overweight (and I am not tall at 5'6"), I was still able to reduce my body weight by about 10% employing some easy strategies discussed above (from 157 down to a lean 141). My body fat is about 15%, which is quite low (recognizing that the examination of body fat is part of another chapter in another book at some other time).

Supplements

I consume, and am a strong advocate of, fish oil, CoQ10, nattokinase, magnesium and another group of herbs, herbal extracts, and plant enzymes (Herbal Cardiovascular Formula) that I mentioned above just briefly. These herbs, extracts and enzymes are not exactly in the category of controlling irregular heartbeats per se, but they are excellent for enhancing cardiovascular health. There is a brief description of the ingredients of these agents in the box below.

Bromelain, Curcumin, Ginger and Gugulipid

The following herbs, herbal extracts and plant enzymes are recommended in the context of heart health for a number of reasons, not the least of which is to act as a natural anti-inflammatory. Many experts feel that much of your body's ailments stem from some sort of inflammation, whether the inflammation is in your joints, your organs or your skin. Just because you do not see the inflammation does not mean it is not there.

Bromelain is a mixture of certain sulfur-containing plant enzymes (in the trade they are called *proteolytic enzymes*, which is the breakdown of proteins into simpler, soluble substances such as peptides and amino acids, as occurs during digestion). Bromelain is obtained from the stem of the pineapple plant. Bromelain is a natural muscle relaxant so I take it to calm my heart muscle as a preventative measure and when it is in an agitated state, ripe for arrhythmias to occur.

Remember the discussion of blood clotting and thrombolytic enzymes in the section dealing with nattokinase? Well, fibrinogen is another component of blood involved in the clotting process. Fibrinogen hinders your blood flow and oxygen delivery by deforming red blood cells, causing red cell aggregation, and thickening the blood by increasing its viscosity, all of which leads to diminished circulation. It binds your blood platelets together, thus causing abnormal blood clot formation in your arteries. Fibrinogen is then converted to fibrin, which is the final step in the blood clotting process.

Fibrinogen contributes to atherosclerosis by incorporating itself into arterial plaque. Along with LDL cholesterol, fibrinogen works to help generate atherosclerotic plaques after fibrinogen initiates the process. Fibrinogen is converted into fibrin, which serves as a base for LDL cholesterol in the formation of the atherosclerotic plaques that can slowly block your arteries.

High levels of fibrinogen can predispose you to coronary and cerebral artery disease, even when other known risk factors such as cholesterol are normal. High fibrinogen levels are at least as great a predictor of cardiovascular disease as any other known risk factor such as elevated LDL cholesterol, elevated triglycerides, high blood pressure, obesity, and diabetes. Fibrinogen levels are high in persons with a family history of heart disease. The predisposition to high fibrinogen levels is genetically inherited, which suggests that fibrinogen may be the genetic factor that causes familial heart disease. Bromelain breaks down that nasty fibrinogen, which was discussed in the previous section, so that the fibrin can be metabolized normally.

There are a number of compounds in your body that initiate the formation of blood clots and the constriction of your blood vessels. These compounds are called *thromboxane*. Ginger is an herb that is a potent inhibitor of blood clot forming synthesis. The beauty of ginger is that it stimulates the production of a substance called *prostacylin*, which inhibits abnormal blood clots in your body.

Ginger also increases the contractile strength of your heart. Scientists call ginger a *"cardiotonic agent"* because of its ability to increase ATP energy production in your heart and to enhance calcium pumping within your heart's cells that is required for optimal cardiac output.

The herbs discussed above (bromelain and ginger) can be obtained individually in health stores and health food departments in certain grocery and drug stores. But, a good product that contains these substances is called Herbal Cardiovascular Formula, produced all together by the nonprofit Life Extension Foundation out of Ft. Lauderdale, Florida. The formula also contains two other heart healthy ingredients, notably curcumin and gugulipid (which are not directly related to palpitations and arrhythmias).

Curcumin is a powerful anti-oxidant and anti-inflammatory. It helps prevent your blood platelets from clumping and is a surprisingly strong supplement in helping suppress viruses. Curcumin can also help you keep your blood platelets healthy,

Gugulipid can act as an antioxidant and help you to maintain normal cholesterol levels and blood platelet function. Its primary action, however, is in maintaining your liver's metabolism of low-density lipoproteins.

I also take other supplements, which are beyond the scope of this book on heart health. So, I am sure you will ask, why don't I eliminate the palpitations totally if I can. Well, my answer is that it is indeed possible, but there are other lifestyle interferences that tend to preclude the complete achievement of that goal. What does this mean?

Exercise

Well, it means that if you are like me, there are certain things in life that you simply like to do or must do to enjoy life to the fullest. And, some of the things that are part of my personal regimen to achieve a healthy as well as enjoyable lifestyle can interfere or otherwise conflict with obtaining a situation where there will be no palpitations. A good example is exercise. I used to lift weights several times per week. However, weight training places a tremendous strain on your heart and I would struggle (meaning that I would have palpitations) most of the time that I would go to the gym. True, breathing properly while going through my reps was helpful, but the fact remains that the weight lifting would normally trigger PVCs and on one occasion caused AFIB. My quandary was that I enjoyed weight training but I definitely did not enjoy palpitations. So, I modified my workout regimen to eliminate heavy weight training and instead I now do strength training without heavy weights, such as pull-ups, push-ups, tricep push ups, and sit ups – and it really helps. Frequently, I will use a machine that essentially uses your own weight as your resistance. Other times I will use a machine that is a "reverse gravity" machine that when you add weight, it actually lightens your load so to speak. Anyway, the bottom line is that I use light weight resistance as my strength training. For cardiovascular training, I use a treadmill primarily, with occasional use of the stair-stepper and the elliptical machine. Typically, I limit cardio to about 30 minutes. And, last but not least, I walk outside in the sunlight whenever possible for about 30-45 minutes.

Food Sensitivities

Another issue is the matter of food sensitivities. I am sensitive to garlic, dairy, chocolate, tomatoes and corn. But, since garlic is almost impossible to avoid I try to cope as much as possible. As far as dairy, I am not only lactose intolerant but the dairy triggers the palpitations as well. But, my morning regimen includes a small one-third cup of organic, lactose-free milk to allow a super-food concoction that I consume daily to taste nice and "creamy" (this is described more particularly immediately below under "Eating Regimen"). Generally, this small amount of dairy is insufficient to cause any real problems.

Eating Regimen

Since I started on the following general eating regimen (I dislike using the "diet" cliché), I have lost about 10% of my starting body weight, which is not bad. I could probably lose more if I wanted to, but my metabolism is sufficiently active so I don't have to engage in much restriction. For breakfast, I rarely eat eggs (and if I do, it's organic brown eggs), and never eat bacon, pork sausage, ham, potatoes, biscuits, cereals of any kind, donuts (shudder the thought), or other breakfast pastries. Typically, I will have a glass of freshly squeezed orange juice about three times a week or so along with 3 PGX™ pills (more particularly described below). When I am not having juice I will take the pills with spring water (in my home city we are benefited from a supplier of fresh water "delivered to my door" that has the highest amount of oxygen of any other supplier). Then, I will eat an apple, pear, strawberries, blueberries, or a combination of all or some of these fruits, along with a home-made, very healthy, and oh so tasty, blueberry bran muffin or oat bran muffin. As your reward for buying this book, I am going to give you my recipe for the best, not to mention healthiest, blueberry bran muffins you will ever eat:

2 cups of whole wheat flour (ideally organic flour)

2 cups of wheat bran (ideally organic wheat bran)

2 level teaspoons of baking soda

2 level teaspoons of baking powder

1 egg (ideally, an organic brown egg) (use 2 eggs if you like a more cake like consistency of the muffin)

1 cup of Agave nectar (this is my secret sweetening ingredient that comes from cactus, which adds a very pleasant sweet taste and has a very low glycemic index (see box below). You can usually pick up Agave nectar at the heath food store or through the Internet.

One-third cup of TheraSweet™ brand sweetener (this is discussed in Part II, Chapter 10, the section entitled "Do Not Continue to Eat Like You Do") below. If you want to substitute Agave for TheraSweet™ just add about two more ounces of Agave.

2/3 of a cup of fat free organic milk

4 tablespoons of Macadamia Nut Oil (best obtained at the health food store or on the Internet)

1 1/3 of a cup of spring water (add more or less spring water as necessary to get a nice smooth consistency, but not too thick)

1/2 of a cup of blueberries (about 30+ blueberries) (fresh or frozen, depending on the season)

Mix all the ingredients together, pour into cupcake papers to be placed in a cupcake or muffin baking pan. Bake at 350 degrees for 23-30 minutes (give or take a few minutes depending on how large you make your muffins). This usually yields me at least 12 medium size muffins. Check around 23 minutes and see how it's baking.

They are the best tasting, healthiest, muffins you ever had. The real beauty of them is they are not made with any processed sugar and they taste just as sweet and delicious as any muffin you ever had. Even more important is the glycemic index of its main sweetening ingredients (Agave and TheraSweet™) are very low.

What is the Glycemic Index

The glycemic index measures how fast a food is likely to raise your blood sugar. It can be a helpful tool in managing your intake blood sugars because it measures how much your blood glucose increases in the two or three hours after eating. It compares foods gram for gram of carbohydrate. Carbohydrates that breakdown quickly during digestion have the highest glycemic indexes. The blood glucose response is fast and high. Carbohydrates that break down slowly, releasing glucose gradually into the blood stream, have low glycemic indexes. The significance of eating foods with a low glycemic index is that you will have a smaller rise in blood glucose levels after meals, have an easier time losing weight, improve your body's sensitivity to insulin, more efficiently help re-fuel carbohydrate stores after exercise, improve diabetes control, keep you fuller for longer, be able to prolong physical endurance.

The numbers reflective of a food's glycemic index is based on glucose, which is one of the fastest carbohydrates available. In other words, glucose is given an arbitrary value of 100 and other carbs are given a number relative to glucose. Faster carbs (higher numbers) are great for raising low blood sugars and for covering brief periods of intense exercise. Slower carbs (lower numbers) are helpful for preventing overnight drops in the blood sugar and for long periods of exercise. As an example, the traditional sugar that is used in most baked goods is "off the charts" in terms of glycemic index.

Examples of high glycemic index foods would be instant rice (124), Corn Flakes™ (119), Rice Krispies™ (117), jellybeans (114), French fries (107), soda crackers (106), potato (boiled/mashed) (104), white bread (100), melba toast (100). couscous (93), ice cream (87), oatmeal (one minute oats) (87), digestive cookies (84), table sugar (sucrose) (83).

Examples of lower glycemic index foods would be popcorn (58). oat bran bread (68), oatmeal (slow cook oats) (70), parboiled rice (68), pumpernickel bread (66), All-Bran™ (60), sweet potato (54), skim milk (46), pasta (40 to 70), Lentils/kidney/baked beans (40 to 69), apple/banana/plum (34 to 69).*

Source: Canadian Diabetes Association

Also for breakfast, I have a LivingFuel™ shake. They are the same folks who created TheraSweet™ but this powdered drink is the best I have ever seen (not to mention tasted), since it is just about the only protein drink that has no soy protein, along with no wheat, dairy, whey, hydrogenated oils, gluten, yeast, fillers or any of that stuff. It just has plenty of flavor (I like their Super Berry flavor), fiber, vitamins, minerals, probiotics, special antioxidants, essential fatty acids and much more. This shake is actually a food substitute that the formulator claims is an "optimized super-food meal replacement." I mix it in a blender with a sliced pre-frozen banana (for thickness and some extra potassium), along with just about 1 cup of spring water and 1/3 of a cup of organic fat free and lactose free milk.

For lunch and dinner, I will have more traditional meals, but I will stay away from the following foods: white potatoes, white bread, white rice, sugar (inclusive of high fructose corn syrup and other high glycemic foods and sugar substitutes), and any processed meat. I try to avoid beef and chicken at traditional food stores and restaurants because of the excruciatingly terrible breeding conditions of those animals. I will always look for free range or natural chicken. If cooking at home, I will prepare natural grass fed buffalo (bison) instead of beef. My intake of fish has been frustratingly reduced in a significant way. I will have fish two times a week and I will avoid farm raised salmon, swordfish and halibut. I usually eat wild Alaskan salmon (when in season), as well as trout (rainbow and ruby red), tilapia, striped bass and Lake Victoria perch.

But, here is the real key to losing weight and treating your body better – don't eat carbohydrates after dinner! No cakes, ice cream, candy, cookies, donuts, or muffins. And, try to skip the chocolate explosion, tiramisu and crème brulee for dessert when you are eating out as well. I know it's hard to resist, but typically you have eaten a big dinner and there should be no reason for you to have the nutritional and physiological need for the sweets other than a psychological craving or even addiction. Remember, these desserts are made to sound and look appetizing, but they have absolutely, positively no nutritional value and can only harm you and your heart (amongst other organs). If you have to eat something because you are famished, have some protein, like a piece of chicken or have some nuts, which is satisfying and filling. And, if you absolutely need something sweet, munch on a nice sweet apple or pear – but, really limit it to one or two bites.

Stress and Lifestyle

I frequently engage in deep breathing (as outlined above) and listen to self-hypnosis tapes on relieving stress. I try to drink plenty of water – when I can remember to do it – and work hard to get enough sleep, although that is the most difficult part of the entire process for me. It is the number one cause of palpitations in my situation. But, I find that walking outside (for about 30-45 minutes) in as much sunlight as the clouds will allow, goes a long way in relieving stress, but also lowering blood pressure which is a symptom of high levels of stress. And, I do not use commercial sunscreen.

When I Have Symptoms of Irregular Heartbeats

When I seem to have palpitations that seem to be occurring with some degree of regularity I will engage in a certain protocol. This is done when I am having them more frequent than two or three times a day. Remember, everyone is different. You might get them as frequent as once every five minutes or sometimes more frequent (even every minute or every 10 or twenty seconds). This does not happen that often, but it may happen to you. In fact, the degree to which arrhythmias can be bothersome differs from individual to individual. The fact of the matter is that most people who get them don't like them and they want to eliminate them or minimize them.

As for me, I first take a deep "cleansing" breath to let some extra oxygen in. Then, I will determine if I am overdue for some of the anti-arrhythmia supplements (I described above). If I am, I will take some omega-3 fish oil, magnesium and Herbal Cardiovascular Formula. Sometimes, I might take two pills of fish oil and Herbal Cardiovascular Formula. Rather than panicking, I will sit down in a comfortable chair and utilize some of the breathing techniques mentioned above. And, I will start to consume some water (at least three cups). If it does not go away by then, I will try to walk outside, but if that is not possible, then I will walk at a slow pace indoors in as large an area as I can find (but, I am careful to make sure that the palpitations are not a prelude to AFIB; if the walking does not help, I sit down and try to relax). Interspersed between all of the above, I will engage in some stress relieving tapping exercises on my head, chest and wrists (EFT technique). I also might take a vitamin B complex pill, as vitamin B has been known to alleviate stress. After a short while (due to the increased consumption of liquids), I will have to urinate once or twice and that actually goes a long way in relieving some of the symptoms.

Having a blood pressure machine is also useful in monitoring your pressure and pulse so you can track your improvement or worsening condition. I have found that increased blood pressure and pulse ratings are often directly related to increased palpitations. When my palpitations subside, my blood pressure goes down and seeing this in print is quite relieving. However, an occasional palpitation once of twice a day is not bothersome.

PART II
Keeping Your Heart Healthy – Period

Introduction to Part II

Part II of *Keeping Your Heart in Rhythm* is really a form of bonus because it goes beyond just preventing, suppressing and eliminating irregular heartbeats. In other words, part II is not intended only for individuals who have an irregular heartbeat problem. Rather, it contains information on keeping your heart healthy, whether or not you have an arrhythmia problem. After all, an irregular beat is just one of the many things that can go wrong with your heart. And, it would be a disservice to you to only point out those strategies that protect against an irregular beat. The goal here is to not only keep your heart in rhythm, but to keep your heart and your overall cardiovascular system healthy and happy overall – naturally, without the use of drugs and invasive procedures. If this can be accomplished, then the chances of attaining an arrhythmia-free life are much greater.

Chapter 6
Respect Your Heart – No One Else Will Be Doing It For You

"Nature is just enough; but men and women must comprehend and accept her suggestions."

—Antoinette Brown Blackwell

In chapter 6, I will start to go beyond the limited discussion of palpitations and arrhythmias. I will examine the reasons why it is so difficult for you to obtain and maintain cardiovascular health. I will explain what ailments are part of the term "heart disease" and how the many forms of this dreaded disease can actually work together synergistically, absolutely destroying the ability of your heart and body as a whole to work efficiently.

I will explore how big business thrives on causing you to believe you need to satisfy a craving for instantaneous gratification – at the expense of long-term heart health? I will uncover how you are misguided and manipulated through sophisticated (and sometimes highly deceptive) marketing and advertising campaigns. I will discuss how your basic human instincts are being exploited every day to your detriment.

And, to what extent does this manipulation and exploitation bring about all sorts of health related problems for you and everyone else? And, even further, to what extent have you failed to understand what your healthcare system can do for you and cannot do for you? In the most riveting chapter yet, we will examine all of these issues and more.

THE NUMBERS – READ 'EM AND WEEP

According to the Centers for Disease Control and Prevention, 61 million Americans currently suffer from cardiovascular disease. This covers a broad spectrum of disorders, including high blood pressure, coronary heart disease (heart attack and chest pain), stroke, congestive heart failure, and birth defects of the heart and blood vessels.

Every year, heart attacks and stroke cause more than 930,000 deaths in the U.S., accounting for 40% of deaths from all causes and making cardiovascular disease the nation's number-one killer. In fact, to place this problem in a more glaring perspective, someone has some form of heart disease every 30 seconds and death occurs from such an event every minute. Sadly, every other person you know is likely to die of heart disease. While cardiovascular disease primarily kills people aged 65 and older, the incidence of sudden death from heart disease is rising in people aged 15 to 34.

Not very surprisingly, the Centers for Disease Control and Prevention has stated that if all types of heart disease were eliminated, Americans would live an average of almost seven years longer.

FALSE ASSUMPTIONS AND MISGUIDED PRIORITIES

Earlier in this book I noted that the human heart is one of the hardest working organisms known to man. Your heart goes and goes, beating non-stop, 24 hours a day, every day of your life. It does not ask for much, other than some decent nutrition and some regular exercise. Instead, most Americans feed their heart (and the rest of their body) everything from toxic tobacco smoke, to excessive alcohol, to artery clogging trans fats from cakes, cookies, crackers, snack foods, vegetable shortenings and some margarines, to white breads and sugars, to foods laced with excessive sodium (salt) and to fried foods. And, on top of that, most Americans find much more pleasure from eating these foods than exercising their heart, because the pleasant taste of sugary and fatty foods is considered to be quite pleasurable. The present experience of exercise, however, is woefully viewed as being painful – being out of breath, having muscles ache, and simply undergoing intense physical labor. Again, one's frame of reference is the present, and the future is only an afterthought for many. They cannot bridge the gap and consider the energizing and stress-reducing future results of basic exercise. After all, as long as their heart does not hurt or does not cause them pain in some manner, then their attention is focused on something more pressing that might provide some other instant gratification.

In short, their heart is taken for granted. Many people assume that when there is a problem, they can go to the doctor and they can be "fixed." They simply expect that their body could very well break down in some manner and expect the doctor, who is a by-product of modern conventional medical science, to cure the problem.

However, there is simply no guarantee about how, or even if, your body will react positively to any course of medical protocol or medication recommended by your doctor. Sadly, your expectations, in terms of what the traditional medical community can do for you after a problem develops, result in frustration, disappointment and falsity – particularly if you rely totally on your physician to solve your health problems. In many cases, you are left with invasive and surgical procedures that are costly, time-consuming, life changing, and downright risky.

As for your heart from a prevention perspective, typically your doctor will tell you to lose weight, improve your eating habits and start exercising. But, they cannot make you do anything unless you are willing. If you do not change your lifestyle, those unhealthy habits lead to symptoms of pain and/or something being wrong. That is when you go to your doctor for help. Once at the doctor's office you will undergo some questioning and some tests. If this investigation reveals a problem, you will be treated, which almost always means that you will be given a prescription for expensive medication. You have a preconceived notion that if you get a prescription for a pill from your doctor, the pill will make things go away. But, sometimes the pills work and sometimes they don't. When they don't, you typically will undergo more tests, usually more sophisticated and complicated than the first ones. Often, these tests show that you need surgery or some type of invasive procedure.

The circuitry and/or structural aspects of your heart may have to be significantly reconfigured in an unnatural manner, only to keep you alive. You then may be placed on strong drugs that cause demonstrable alterations of your biochemical make-up, all with serious side effects, which can be quite inconvenient and painful, in and of themselves. Mechanical devices, such as artificial valves, pacemakers and defibrillators may have to be placed near or even in your heart.

Sadly, what we call modern medicine is really treatment for the damage that has already been done.

If you are an individual with an irregular heartbeat that is classified as harmless or benign, you know how terribly disconcerting and uncomfortable it can be – and this is when you do not have inherent heart disease. So, just imagine how awful it must be to have heart disease, where the organ, that pumps your blood to all other organs non-stop and keeps you alive, is in a significant state of repair and disarray. It is terribly unfortunate that people are so accepting of the inevitability of their heart disease.

While there are a lot of very good doctors in the traditional medical community, the treatment and cure of serious heart disease still has a long way to go. With heart disease as the number #1 killer in America as of the date of this writing, there simply cannot be enough knowledge and preventative efforts taken by all Americans.

We are all facing an uphill battle with respect to fighting heart disease. Our healthcare system is totally preoccupied with merely the diagnosis, treatment and cure of disease rather than prevention; our drug companies are more concerned with profits than safety; and our hospitals are making too much money on heart problems, not to mention the problem of having to delicately balance quality treatment against reducing the risks of litigation; and our doctors are all too often schooled on pushing drugs rather than natural prevention and healing.

After all, the money in medicine is in cardiac care and surgery. The tab of treating ailing hearts in this country approaches $300 billion a year in the U.S. – about 20% of the health-care economy! About $30 billion is spent on cardiovascular drugs alone. With roughly 15 million Americans suffering from heart disease and tens of millions more burdened by high blood pressure or high cholesterol, treating heart disease has become an industry. More than a thousand hospitals offer full-service heart programs. They typically account for more than 20% of hospital revenues and sometimes 50% of profits. Indeed, heart surgery is what keeps hospitals in business. Cardiac care is unquestionably profitable.

AN UPHILL BATTLE

And, it does not end there. The food products in your grocery stores are mostly loaded with sugars, trans fats and/or simple carbohydrates, not to mention being over-processed and over-preserved. Your fruits and your vegetables are being increasingly genetically modified so that they can become more disease resistant, not to mention being laced with chemical fertilizers, herbicides and pesticides so that your farmers can produce crops that are more efficiently and more profitably distributed. Much of the meats you eat are from animals infused with antibiotics and growth hormones (so that they can be bred quickly, profitably and with the least amount of disease despite being raised in traditionally unsanitary and sometimes inhumane conditions. Your dairy products are pasteurized and homogenized (which on its face has a very protective sound). But, in reality the milk is heated at very high temperatures killing all the beneficial enzymes in it, and being homogenized, it completely compromises the chemical structure of the milk's molecules so that when you consume the milk, it damages your arteries (further contributing to atherosclerosis) and causes digestive problems. And, as you have read in Chapter 5, your fish (in most cases) are loaded with either toxic chemicals, mercury, PCBs, antibiotics, hormones or a combination of all of them. And, this does not even cover your processed foods, which will be further discussed in this Part II, in boxes, cans and jars that prejudice your health even further.

Simply stated, your food is not the same as it was when you were younger. Today, your food is full of toxins that kill the beneficial enzymes, eliminating much of the nutritional value. The food you eat is so mechanically altered it actually becomes man-made foreign substances that your body really cannot handle. In short, it is virtually impossible to go to the grocery store and purchase food that is not loaded with chemicals, significantly depleted of nutritional value, and energetically altered.

Your restaurants seem to be the real killers – sacrificing health for taste by overwhelming their food with salt, non-organic butters, and extremely unhealthy (but, of course, ever so tasty) sugars and fats. After all, no taste equals no customers, sad as it may be. One can very easily conclude that many of the food products provided through food distribution chains and restaurants are prepared, processed and/or formulated to be addictive rather than nutritious, tasty rather than wholesome and disease promoting rather than disease preventing. The more the large food distributors keep it that way the more you will crave and purchase more food, which in turn means more profits for them.

And, the list goes on topped off with our federal, state and local Governments still allowing the sale of cigarettes, one of the top causes of heart disease. The paradox is that Governments are supposed to protect taxpayers and tax revenues are supposed to accomplish that goal. The ultimate paradox is that the monies obtained through tax revenues are the result of a consumable (cigarettes) that does exactly the opposite of what Governments are supposed to do.

Big business will do just about anything to make their products cheaper and more profitable. Again, profits at the expense of health and safety are the prime mover.

It is amazing that so many people in this country can be so intelligent and have such common sense. When the issue of food and the other products that people physically consume enters into the equation, they throw "caution to the wind", so to speak. They disregard the true needs of their bodies and succumb to the temptations of instant gratification. Most Americans have been programmed to view food more as entertainment rather than essential fuel that their body needs to keep running properly.

THE CONSEQUENCES OF OUR OWN INACTION

One of the most profound and overlooked secrets to lasting, pain-free and robust health is a healthy circulatory system. This is because your entire system depends on a continuous supply of oxygen to every corner of your body. Cut this supply off and you would die in a matter of minutes. Ever have your feet feel numb? It is because they are not getting the oxygen they need. Your arteries are the "delivery route" over which this life-giving substance travels. If these pathways are blocked or narrowed, your body starts to gasp for what little oxygen it can get. Your body has to work harder and harder to do the simplest tasks. The condition is like someone holding a pillow to your face.

The medical term for this condition is "*atherosclerosis*", which is commonly called hardening of the arteries. It is a gradual, dynamic inflammatory condition where your arteries become narrow and stiff and blood flow to and from your heart is blocked to a certain extent, and takes many years to develop. Until that time and even when the disease results, you have no pain. So, most people "let it slide", so to speak, whether for budgetary reasons or reasons of denial.

Atherosclerosis is characterized by the build-up of yellowish plaque in the narrow inner opening in your arteries through which blood flows. This plaque consists of fatty substances called lipids, which further consist of cholesterol, calcium, cellular waste products and fibrin, that blood clotting material I have referred to several times. As the plaque builds and grows, your artery walls become thicker, and partially or totally clog the pathways of the blood flow to and from your heart. When your blood vessel pathways are healthy, they are smooth and slick like a well-oiled surface; conversely, when your blood vessel walls are unhealthy, they are sticky and plaque naturally attaches itself to the vessel walls and atherosclerosis sets in.

This condition is bad enough, but it can get worse when this layer of plaque breaks off (typically after it gets large and brittle) where two things can happen.

First, when the layer of plaque breaks off a blood clot develops to seal the break. This can have the further effect of an even greater degree of narrowing of your arteries and reducing the amount of blood that can pass through. When your heart has to work harder, due to the plaque build up, it becomes enlarged. When it becomes bigger like this, it is more difficult to maintain blood flow and enough oxygen to your cells. You feel tired, cannot perform physical activity very well. More serious heart disease is just around the corner. More specifically, if the blockage partially or completely deprives your heart of enough oxygen, a heart attack (also known as *myocardial infarction*) can result. Your heart continues to beat, but the cells in your heart begin to die. The more time that passes without treatment, the greater the damage. How do you know if you're having a heart attack? Well, if you have discomfort (in the form of uncomfortable pressure, pain or squeezing) in the center of your chest and lasts for a short while, or goes away and comes back, you may be having a heart attack. Actually, you can have pain in your back, neck, jaw or stomach and it can be a sign of a heart attack. Shortness of breath, nausea and lightheadedness are additional signs of problems. But, even if a blood clot does not occur, excessive plaque can cause a response called a "vasospasm" in the artery, which has the effect of impeding blood flow and depriving your heart of oxygen.

Eerily, heart disease is a slow, silent killer. People may think of the amorphous term "blockages", but it does not give true meaning to the silent destructive power of calcium plaque build-up and cholesterol deposits choking your blood vessels. In the tiniest amounts, they quietly build up and up. Your entire system slows down, so doing anything requires double the effort. This cannot only cause a heart attack or stroke, but it can affect your vision, sex life, joints, memory, cholesterol level, energy level, and much more.

When people hear the term "plaque" they most likely think of the sticky stuff that clings to your teeth and your dental hygienist can scrape off at your next cleaning. In the context of heart problems, a similar build-up of solid residue occurs but it is not just isolated in the heart muscle. Plaque and cholesterol can form anywhere in your entire circulatory system, including many areas where surgery cannot reach. Poor circulation will affect oxygen delivery to every cell, tissue, gland and system connected to your circulatory system. This includes your lungs, sexual organs, kidneys and legs. But, it has different names.

Hypertension or high blood pressure is just one of the consequences of atherosclerosis. There can be coronary heart disease, which results from the partial blockages of blood flow and a resultant lack of oxygen getting to the heart. The lack of oxygen getting to your heart is called *ischemia*. This will often happen after exercise, physical exertion or stress. A heart attack is sometimes the culmination of full-blown coronary heart disease. A significant degree of *ischemia* can cause a heart attack or cardiac arrest, where your heart suddenly stops beating. Other signs of coronary heart disease are various types of irregular heartbeats, angina pains or shortness of breath.

We learned about arrhythmias in part I, but *angina* is a different animal, where there is mild to severe chest pain resulting from not enough oxygen getting to the heart. Sometimes your angina pain happens as expected. Other times it comes and goes in an unpredictable manner. Whatever the delivery mode, if you have a severe squeezing, suffocating, or burning feeling that is located under the breastbone, it can be angina. It can even spread to your left shoulder and wrist as well as into your teeth and jaw area. You may even feel numb or have a loss of sensation in those areas.

As you get older you have to work harder at preventing plaque buildup and heart disease. This is because as you get older, your arteries become stiffer, the heart walls thicken, and the heart muscle does not necessarily contract and relax as it once did. The heart slowly loses its pumping capacity and works less efficiently. Again, taking the condition of your heart for granted over the years, and not taking affirmative steps to keep your cardiovascular system clean, can result in your developing a condition known as *"congestive heart failure."* This involves your heart not pumping enough blood in relation to the amount returning to the lungs. Your blood gets accumulated in your veins. This results in your lungs filling with fluid or swelling of your feet and legs. Symptomatically, you will frequently have difficulty breathing and you also may be tired more than normal. Other manifestations may be a dry cough, persistent cold or wheezing. Congestive heart failure also is a telltale sign of more serious problems such as atherosclerosis and heart valve problems.

When your brain is impacted, by insufficient oxygen to the brain, it's called a *stroke*. This condition, which is the third leading killer of Americans, is discussed in greater detail in chapter 9, but suffice it to say at this point, that there is a great deal of misunderstanding amongst most people as to what a stroke is all about or what causes it. Most people think that a stroke is a random occurrence that cannot be controlled. This is not the case, as most strokes are preventable.

Strokes can occur in two ways. This first way is really not in the context of heart related problems. This involves bleeding in your brain by means of a blood vessel bursting causing intense pressure in the skull area. The affected area of your brain can then drown or die from the pressure. This is the most deadly form of stroke and the only good news is that it happens in the minority of cases of the disease – about 20%.

The other 80% occur from clogged blood vessels in your brain. Blood cannot get though to your brain because the vessels are too narrow from plaque build-up or because a clot blocks the passage. If oxygen-rich blood cannot get through to a part of your brain, brain tissue dies and that area's brain functions or memories are lost. And, once you suffer a stroke you are more likely to suffer another. But, the process starts long before you suffer this damage. It begins with reducing the build-up of plaque.

If you're thinking, "I am fine as I don't have any pain and am feeling good", think again. The average 20-year old eating a typical American young adult fast food regimen typically has a 20% closure of three important coronary arteries already. Deadly plaque is dangerous because it sneaks up on you without warning – and then it strikes. Most people think they are fine, until they get the shock of their lives.

Just remember, when you chomp down on those fried chicken fingers, fries and some nice apple pie (and even if you do eat a bit healthier than that), and after you have just let another week go by without much exercise, coronary heart disease is the single biggest killer of men and women in America. Over 6 million people are hospitalized each year with a health problem due to cardiovascular issues. And, ever so worrisome, 50% of men and 64% of women who die of this disease have no previous symptoms.

YOU MUST BE PROACATIVE

The problem with most people is their assumption that no symptoms and no pain equate with no problems. And, if there is pain, all they need do is go to their doctor for the appropriate corrective measures. Unfortunately for these people that is the most incorrect assumption of their lives.

You really need to go beyond what your physician (whose abilities are all too often overrated) tells you. It is indeed rare for your doctor to do anything other than prescribe some expensive drugs (with terrible side effects) or risky invasive procedures. It is a rare doctor who lays out a plan of natural and safe nutritional supplements, inclusive of herbs, as aids or cures.

Largely, it is up to you to educate yourself about natural alternatives and the very positive side effects of those alternatives. You simply cannot rely upon advances by the mainstream medical community to eliminate heart disease. Your good health depends upon you taking positive action. However, taking positive action is no easy task, particularly in light of the state of our health care system (that has many other agendas besides prevention and cure) and the state of the food service and food distribution industry (which too heavily focuses on profits, cost savings and consumer taste rather than nutrition).

But, the good news is that a healthier heart is within your reach. If you are willing to take positive action, such as a better diet, supplements of vitamins, minerals and herbs, more physical exercise and weight management, as well as certain lifestyle changes, you can prevent and even fight heart disease and win the battle and experience the pleasure that peace of mind brings.

So, what can be done proactively to keep your heart healthy and enjoy life to the fullest extent possible? The next three chapters in Part II lay out a basic plan of personal preventative healthcare – naturally – so that heart disease and heart related problems, with its attendant drugs, invasive procedures and surgery, can potentially be out of your lifetime picture. So, the first thing to focus on is to simply follow the suggestions discussed in Chapter 5 above, notably the "Seven Natural and Safe Ways to Protect Against Irregular Heatbeats."

Irregular heartbeat or no irregular heartbeat, you owe it to yourself to engage in these lifestyle changes. Specifically, take fish oil and nattokinase to reduce the blood clotting protein fibrinogen and inhibit platelet aggregation, which in turn prevents blood-clot formation on active, ruptured coronary plaque that would otherwise result in a heart attack. Reduce stress by drinking more water, breathing better, and taking courses in meditation and yoga. Lower blood pressure and insure all of your enzymes work for you (rather than against you) by taking magnesium, nattokinase and CoQ10 daily – and, once again, drink plenty of water. Strengthen your heart, exercise longer, feel and breathe better, and suffer less build up of fluid in the legs by taking CoQ10. And lastly, take fish oil and nattokinase to cleanse your arteries, decrease cholesterol, and increase your oxygen delivery and bioavailability of other nutrients.

Chapter 7
Avoid Trans Fat At All Costs

"The quality of your life is dependent upon the quality of the life of your cells. If the bloodstream is filled with waste products, the resulting environment does not promote a strong, vibrant, healthy cell life – nor a biochemistry capable of creating a balanced emotional life for an individual."

—Anthony Robbins

So, what else can we do to become heart healthy? Well, the first place to start is to examine an area that has been targeted as the culprit for much of the heart disease problems that we face today and for years to come. We will take a long hard look at trans fats. I will tell you where trans fats come from and what happens to them in your body. After I am done, you may never eat a cookie, cracker, donut, cake, pie, fried food, microwave popcorn, or margarine again. And, we will see how saturated fats have been unfairly blamed for much of the problems that trans fats, and even some polyunsaturated fats, have caused. I will also submit to you the real culprits for the problems that saturated fats have been long blamed for.

In Chapter 7, I will describe what fats are supposed to do for you, and the different kinds of fats. You will be surprised to learn how the oils from fats are manufactured and what actually happens to the oils that you consume on an everyday basis. I will describe how "free radicals" are formed and how they can have such a ruinous impact on your heart health. On the other hand, there are some simple rules to follow that can stop, and even potentially reverse, the slow and silent advance of atherosclerotic plaque and the lurking, and potentially deadly, correlated cardiovascular consequences.

FATS IN GENERAL

We continually hear of fat being something bad or something we should avoid for the most part. However, all fat is not bad, as we need fat to survive. Fat is a major source of energy for the body and aids in the absorption of vitamins A, D, E, and K and carotenoids. Both animal and plant-derived food products contain fat, and when eaten in moderation, fat is important for proper growth, development, and maintenance of good health. As a food ingredient, fat provides taste, consistency, and stability and helps you feel full. In addition, parents should be aware that fats are an especially important source of calories and nutrients for infants and toddlers (up to 2 years of age), who have the highest energy needs per unit of body weight of any age group.

Most people are under the impression that saturated fats are bad, polyunsaturated fats are good and monounsaturated fats are somewhat of an unknown (although most people would probably classify them as good). This is largely the impression created from advertising and marketing propaganda to which most people are commonly exposed. So, let's examine each of these fats in detail and determine what they are comprised of and how they are created. The effort here is to arrive at what I consider to be the truth about each of these fats and their impact on your heart health.[25]

FATS AND ESSENTIAL FATTY ACIDS

Fats and oils are mixtures of fatty acids. Essential fatty acids are nutrients we must have to stay healthy. Each fat or oil is designated "saturated," "monounsaturated" or "polyunsaturated," depending on what type of fatty acid predominates.

Saturated fatty acids

The key elemental ingredients of essential fatty acids are hydrogen and carbon. Without getting into too much high school chemistry, this type of essential fatty acid has all the hydrogen the carbon atoms can hold. Saturated fats are usually solid at room temperature, and they're more stable – that is, they don't combine readily with oxygen and turn rancid. Some saturated fatty acids can raise blood cholesterol, and when combined with other poor dietary choices can raise the risk of coronary heart disease and stroke. Notice I said "combined with other poor dietary choices." Raising blood cholesterol is not in and of itself that bad unless there is something else bad going on in your body to turn your cholesterol into your enemy.

Monounsaturated fatty acids

Monounsaturated oils are liquid at room temperature but start to solidify at refrigerator temperatures. For example, salad dressing containing olive oil turns cloudy when refrigerated but is clear at room temperature. Monounsaturated fatty acids seem to lower blood cholesterol when substituted for saturated fats.

Polyunsaturated fatty acids

Polyunsaturated oils, which contain mostly polyunsaturated fatty acids, are liquid at room temperature and in the refrigerator. They easily combine with oxygen in the air to become rancid. However, polyunsaturated fatty acids help lower total blood cholesterol when substituted for saturated fats.

While unsaturated fats (monounsaturated and polyunsaturated) and even many saturated fats may be all right from the standpoint of heart health (as compared with other types of disease prevention) when consumed in moderation, trans fats are not. Saturated fat can, and trans fat does, increase a particular type of cholesterol level in the blood (it's called LDL cholesterol, which I will describe in more detail below). But, saturated fat increases it for a specific reparative reason (again, which I will describe in more detail below). It is advisable to choose foods low in, or not having, trans fat and foods that do not raise this LDL cholesterol as part of a healthful diet. In fact, even many polyunsaturated fats, they way they are currently processed can actually cause all sorts of bodily breakdowns, much to the surprise of many who historically believed that the low cholesterol, low saturated fat (high in polyunsaturated fat) diet was the best.

So, what is all this notoriety about trans fats and what is its impact on your cardiovascular system?

CAUTION: NOT ALL SATURATED FATS ARE BAD AND NOT ALL POLYUNSATURATED FATS AND OILS ARE GOOD

Most Americans, as well as most people around the world, generally assume that heart disease results from the consumption of an excessive amount of saturated fats and cholesterol. However, you would be surprised to learn that there is, in fact, very little evidence to support the contention that a diet low in cholesterol and saturated fat actually reduces death from heart disease or in any way increases one's life span.[26]

If you take a look over the last fifty years, the consumption of butter and animal fats have actually declined! It is further notable that during the same period, the consumption of sugar, processed foods, margarine, shortening and refined oils has skyrocketed. People have been dying, but it has not been from saturated fats and cholesterol. In fact, in a paper prepared by Mary Enig and Sally Fallon, *The Truth About Saturated Fat*, it is reported that studies continuously show that the more a particular group consumed saturated fats, the healthier and longer the life span. What was not eaten by these subjects was vegetable oil, white flour and processed foods.

It is quite interesting that in the early part of the 20th century Americans ate much more saturated and monounsaturated fats from butter, lard, coconut oil and olive oil. Now, the vast majority of oils at the traditional supermarket are derived from soy, corn, canola and safflower. It is submitted that the negativity surrounding saturated fats has been way overrated and the benefits of polyunsaturated fats has been way overstated.

The real problem with saturated fats is that they "hang around" with the wrong set of "friends", so to speak. In other words, it's not the saturated fat in meat that is killing you; it is the omega-6 fatty acids that are doing it. In fact, the way livestock is now raised, there is more of the harmful omega-6 fatty acids in meat than ever before. And, what about fried foods that have saturated fats? It's the saturated fats that always get the bad rap from the marketers of polyunsaturated oils (armed with their hidden agendas). Isn't it odd that trans fats and omega-6 fatty acids most always seem to be at the scene of the alleged cholesterol crime as well?

Saturated Fats

There is hardly any strong evidence that saturated fats are the ones that generate and make up the dangerous plaque that clogs your arteries. In fact, if you examine the fat that actually causes the "clogging", less than 30% is saturated. The rest is unsaturated, most of which is polyunsaturated.

Moreover, these saturated fats exist throughout your entire body naturally, as they constitute about 50% of your cell membranes and are needed to utilize your essential fatty acids. They enhance your immune system and certain types of saturated fatty acids (called the short and medium chain saturated fatty acids) protect you against destructive microorganisms in your digestive tract. In fact, did you know that the fat around your heart muscle is highly saturated, being the preferred food for the heart and in particular, in times of stress!

Your body is capable of synthesizing the saturated fatty acids that it needs from carbohydrates. However, not all saturated fatty acids are the same. There are subtle differences in the various types of saturated fats. Therefore, it is important that you try to vary your intake of these fatty acids – all having different, profound health implications. It is simply unwise for you to have excessive saturated fats or avoid all saturated fats. If you did, you could have serious health consequences.

Polyunsaturated Fats and Oils

Polyunsaturated oils, which include vegetable oils like corn, soy, safflower and canola, are the worst oils to cook with because of the trans-fatty acids introduced during the hydrogenation process, making them highly reactive due to their chemical structure. They become "oxidized" and go rancid easily when heated (with the accompanying oxygen and moisture) and really should not be used in cooking as it gives rise to a tremendous amount of free radical activity.

Oxidation, Free Radicals and Antioxidants

When you think of oxygen I am sure you are thinking of something positive, as oxygen is the key to your existence and without it you could not survive for more than a few minutes. While it is true that oxygen keeps you alive, but at the same time, it can even kill you.

The concept of free radicals and oxidation in your body is the subject of many books and research papers. Suffice it to say, when your body uses oxygen, it allows you to burn glucose and provides you with energy. But, your body produces byproducts through the process of oxidation. These byproducts are called "free radicals." Free radicals create havoc by neutralizing the beneficial chemical processes that occur in your body, and literally causes you to age quicker. You have seen what oxygen does to unprotected metal – it rusts. Well, the same type of reaction is happening in your body when free radicals take their toll. In so doing, free radicals damage the skin to cause wrinkles and premature aging, the tissues and organs to set the stage for tumors, and the blood vessels to initiate the buildup of plaque. Free radicals have been linked with premature aging, arthritis, Alzheimer's disease and numerous other autoimmune diseases. Enig and Fallon, *supra.*

This "oxidative stress" clearly becomes detrimental to your well being, damaging your healthy cells and tissues, inclusive of your arteries. When your bad cholesterol is oxidized it is chemically altered so that it infiltrates your arteries and does some significant damage to the tissues therein.

The way to keep free radicals from damaging your cholesterol and your body as a whole is to zap them with antioxidants. Antioxidants are nutrients that seek out free radicals and destroy them before they can do any more damage to your body. If you want to live a long, healthy, disease-free life as much as possible, you have to consume plenty of antioxidants, particularly in today's society.

Having stated all that, what actually happens in your body to cause this destructive phenomenon? Let's recall your elementary school science class where you certainly learned about molecules, atoms and electrons (which are the building blocks of your cells). Your cells have many, many atoms within the molecules comprising your cells. The oxygen atom in particular has electrons that rotate in pairs around it. When the one electron breaks off, the remaining electron is considered to be "unpaired" and the molecule becomes unstable. This "free radical" atom is formed looking for any electron they can find and in so doing they sabotage other cells. When this occurs other cell structures are destroyed, which in turn causes more free radicals and the destructive cycle is perpetuated. Your tissues are damaged and diseases result.

Vitamins A, C, E, beta carotene and folic acid are excellent antioxidants that destroy the free radicals, as are certain minerals such as selenium. Garlic, grape seed extract and glutathione are also examples of highly beneficial antioxidants.

Alpha lipoic acid is considered by some to be the best antioxidant available to remove an unusually large number of free radicals.

Unfortunately, most of the diets in America involve polyunsaturated fats, such as canola oil, corn oil and safflower oil that contain way too much omega-6 linoleic acid and not enough omega-3 linoleic acid (mainly because it is profitable to market and sell these types of oils). Excess consumption of polyunsaturated oils has been shown to contribute to a large number of diseases, including increased cancer and heart disease (high blood pressure, blood clots, and inflammation), immune system dysfunction, damage to the liver, reproductive organs and lungs; digestive disorders; depressed learning ability, impaired growth, and weight gain. (Enig and Fallon)

But, it must be remembered that not all polyunsaturated fats are bad. The good kind of polyunsaturated oils are from legumes, grains, nuts, green vegetables, fish and olive oil.

The Story of Pritikin

A big advocate of the low-fat, low cholesterol diet was Nathan Pritikin. Actually, Pritikin advocated elimination of sugar, white flour and all processed foods from the diet and recommended the use of fresh raw foods, whole grains and a strenuous exercise program; but it was the low-fat aspects of his regime that received the most attention in the media. People who used the diet found that they had lost weight and that their blood cholesterol levels and blood pressure declined. But Pritikin soon found that the fat-free diet presented many problems, such as people just could not stay on it. Those who possessed enough will power to remain fat-free for any length of time developed a variety of health problems including low energy, difficulty in concentration, depression, weight gain and mineral deficiencies. Pritikin may have not gotten heart disease but his low-fat diet did not prevent him from getting cancer. He died, in the prime of life, of suicide when he realized that his "diet" was not curing his cancer.

THE PROCESSING OF FATS AND OILS – THE OLD AND THE NEW

How the Oil You Eat is Extracted

Many years ago, fruits, nuts and seeds were the foods used to produce the oils and it resulted from using slow stone presses. Nowadays, the seeds that contain this oil are processed in large factories by swiftly crushing them and exposing them to very high temperatures. Then pressure is applied, generating more heat. All the while, the oil is exposed to damaging light and oxygen. But, there is more. Modern day big business needing to maximize its resources to the "last drop" so to speak, and to capture all of the oil from the pulp of the remaining fruit, nut or seed, have their processors treat the residue with a number of chemical solvents, which are not only toxic but they tend to retain the toxic pesticides which were originally on the fruits, seeds and nuts before processing begins. Doesn't that sound appetizing?

In addition to all of that, the high-temperatures that were used during the processing cause the chemical structure of the resultant product to be in a state of disarray, creating a dangerous by-product (resulting from exposing oils to tremendous amounts of heat, light and pressure), notably dangerous "free radicals." In addition, antioxidants, which were contained in the original food product before the extraction began, such as fat-soluble vitamin E, and which protect the body from these damaging free radicals, are either neutralized or destroyed by high temperatures and pressures. In many, but not all cases, additional chemical preservatives (themselves being suspected of causing cancer and brain damage) are added to these oils to replace vitamin E and other natural preservatives destroyed by heat.

Now, let's contrast that with a better, safer, more natural method to extract oils, with the resultant product usually being found in your health food store rather than the mainstream supermarket. Lower temperatures are used and there is minimal exposure to light and oxygen thus preserving the integrity of the fatty acids of the original product. These are known as "expeller pressed" unrefined oils. They will remain fresh for a long time if stored properly in dark bottles and in the case with some oils, stored in the refrigerator.

Where Trans Fats Come From

Trans fats were developed during the backlash against saturated fat – the claimed artery-clogging animal fats found in butter, cream and meats. Then food manufacturers realized that trans fats lasted longer than butter without going rancid. The ultimate consequence of the revelation is that trans fats are found in a large percentage of the products on your supermarket shelves – although luckily that percentage is starting to decline.

Basically, trans fat is made when manufacturers add hydrogen to vegetable oil – a process called hydrogenation.[27] For us laypeople, unlike other fats, the majority of trans fat is formed when food manufacturers turn liquid oils into solid fats like shortening and hard margarine by adding pressure.

A Technical Explanation of Hydrogenation

In a nutshell, hydrogenation is a process by which vegetable oils are converted to solid fats simply by adding hydrogen atoms. All fatty acids are chains of carbon atoms with hydrogen atoms attached. With trans fats, hydrogen atoms are on opposite sides of the chain of carbon atoms at the carbon-carbon double bond. Under high temperatures, these hydrogen atoms change position on the fatty acid chain. Before hydrogenation, pairs of hydrogen atoms occur together on the chain, causing the chain to bend slightly and creating a concentration of electrons at the site of the double bond (which is a configuration most commonly found in nature). With hydrogenation, one hydrogen atom of the pair is moved to the other side so that the molecule straightens. This is called the trans formation, which is rarely found in nature. Trans means "across" in Latin, thus the term "trans fats"

So, why would they do this to perfectly good vegetable oil? The answer is very simple – hydrogenation increases the shelf life and flavor stability of foods containing these fats as well as making the food less greasy tasting. Crackers, for example, can stay on the shelf and stay crispy for years in part because of the hydrogenated fats in them. However, the stiffer and harder fats are, the more they clog up your arteries.

To produce this oil, manufacturers begin with the cheapest oils, such as soy, corn, cottonseed or canola, already rancid from the extraction process described above. They then mix them with tiny metal particles, which in most cases is still another chemical called nickel oxide. Hydrogen gases, high pressures, high temperatures, soap-like emulsifiers and starch are further used to process the oil. Bleach, dyes and flavoring are used to eliminate unpleasant odors, colors and tastes.

Many restaurants use this type of resultant hydrogenated product since they are less expensive than butter and more stable than unsaturated fat. Hydrogenated vegetable oil is often chosen for deep-frying. As noted above, trans fat can be found in vegetable shortenings, some margarines, cookies, pastries, crackers (even healthy sounding ones like Nabisco Wheat Thins), cookies, snack foods, granola bars, chips, salad dressings, many processed foods, and other foods made with or fried in partially hydrogenated oils, such as French fries, fried chicken, and doughnuts.

What Happens to Trans Fats Inside Your Body

Most of these trans fats are toxic to your body, but unfortunately your digestive system does not recognize them as such. Instead of being eliminated, trans fats are incorporated into cells with the result that your cells actually become partially hydrogenated! Once in place, trans fatty acids (with their misplaced hydrogen atoms) create havoc in your cell metabolism because chemical reactions can only take place when electrons in the cell membranes are in certain arrangements or patterns, which the hydrogenation process has disturbed.

Trans fats do the same thing in your body that bacon grease does to kitchen sinks. Over time, they can "clog the pipes" that feed the heart and brain, which can lead to heart attack or stroke risk. There is no useful purpose in the human body of these man-made fats.

Trans fats pose a higher risk of heart disease than saturated fats, which were once believed to be the worst kind of fats. While it is true that saturated fats (found in butter, cheese, beef, coconut and a few other oils) raise total cholesterol levels (again, that in and of itself is not that bad), trans fats go a step further. Trans fats increase blood levels of low density lipoprotein (LDL), or what many people call "bad" cholesterol, which contributes to the build up of fatty plaque in arteries, which in turn increases your risk for heart disease. Trans fats not only raise total cholesterol levels, they also deplete high density lipoprotein (HDL), known as "good" cholesterol, which helps protect against heart disease. Also, it is no surprise that trans fat consumption is one of the major sources of obesity in this country.

To say the same thing a bit differently, trans fats raise LDL cholesterol levels slightly less than do saturated fats but saturated fats also raise levels of high density lipoprotein (HDL) or "good" cholesterol, and trans fatty acids do not. Thus, it is fairly easy to conclude that trans fats are worse.

Trans fats can also cause type 2 diabetes. Researchers at the Harvard School of Public Health in Boston suggest that replacing trans fats in the diet with other fats (such as vegetable oils, salmon, etc.) can reduce diabetes risk by as much as 40%. Altered partially hydrogenated fats are also known to cause other negative effects, such as sexual and immune system dysfunction, birth defects, decreased visual acuity, and a host of other problems.

The FDA estimates that Americans aged 20 and older consume 5.8 grams of trans fats per day – that's about 2.6% of our daily calories. By comparison, we consume 4 to 5 times more saturated fat per day. About 40% of our trans fat intake comes from cakes, cookies, cracker, pies and bread, while 17% comes from margarine.

One problem with the use of trans fat is that food companies, as of the date of this writing, are not required to list it on nutrition labels. So, as a consumer, you have no way of knowing how much trans fat is in the food you are eating. Further, there is no upper safety limit recommended for the daily intake of trans fat. The Food and Drug Administration (FDA) has only said that the "intake of trans fats should be as low as possible."

The FDA has announced a step in the right direction by requiring food manufacturers to list trans fat on Nutrition Facts labels. The bad news is that the labels are not required until 2006, so you, as a consumer, will need to fend for yourself when making food choices until that time.

How To Determine Dangerous Levels of Trans Fat in Foods

While some foods like bakery items and fried foods are obvious sources of trans fat, other processed foods, such as cereals and waffles, can also contain trans fat. One tip to determine the amount of trans fat in your food is to read the ingredient label and look for a listing of "shortening, hydrogenated or partially hydrogenated oil." The higher up on the list these ingredients appear, the more trans fat. Products that contain vegetable shortening may also contain trans fats. You can also add up the amount of fat in a product You can also add up the amount of fat in a product (saturated, monounsaturated and polyunsaturated), provided the amounts are listed, and compare the total with the total fat on the label. If they

don't match up, the difference is likely trans fat, especially if partially hydrogenated oil is listed as one of the first ingredients. Another tip is to watch out for
hydrogenated or partially hydrogenated (soybean, canola, cottonseed or other
oil). Look to see if the hydrogenated oil is in the first 3-4 ingredients. If it is, this
generally means there is a lot of it in the product and you will want to avoid it.

One current deceptive technique food manufacturers employ is to break up
the components of the food (such as coating and the filling). They then take up
half of the ingredient listing with a full description of the first component and its
ingredients, such as the inside filling of the food item, thus camouflaging the second ingredient, often hydrogenated fat, which appears later into the product listing.

Also, don't be fooled by fast food restaurants. The phrase "we cook in vegetable oil" can mean liquid or hydrogenated oil. Even the phrase "no cholesterol
containing all vegetable oil" can be misleading, as vegetable oil can raise your
body's cholesterol if it is a hydrogenated or partly hydrogenated vegetable oil.

In 2003, a lawsuit was filed against Nabisco, the Kraft Foods unit that makes
Oreo cookies, seeking a ban on the sale of Oreo cookies because they contain
trans fat, making them dangerous to eat. The case was later withdrawn because
the lawyer who filed the suit said the publicity surrounding the case accomplished
what he set out to do, notably, create awareness about the dangers of trans fat.
Kraft is also among the companies making efforts to reduce trans fatty acid in
their products.

WHAT KIND OF OILS SHOULD YOU USE

Olive oil is one of the best oils due to its fairly stable nature and low saturated and
omega-6 fat content, amongst other reasons. It contains a high percentage of
oleic acid, which makes olive oil ideal for salads and for cooking at moderate temperatures. Extra virgin olive oil is also rich in antioxidants.

Macadamia nut oil is higher in the monounsaturated fats, which reduces the
risk of heart disease, cancer and diabetes. Moreover, it is very stable at high heat
and tastes great, lending a nice buttery richness to foods.

Peanut oil has a high percentage of omega-6 fatty acids and thus presents a
potential danger, so use of peanut oil should be strictly limited. Sesame oil is
somewhat similar in composition to peanut oil. It can be used for frying because
it contains unique antioxidants that are not destroyed by heat. It also has unique
blood pressure lowering properties.

Safflower, corn, sunflower, soybean and cottonseed oils are also high in omega-6 and are low in omega-3 fatty acids (except soybean oil). As noted above, the use of omega-6 oils in the diet is dangerous. Moreover, these oils are very unstable when heated and their use should essentially be eliminated (there is an exception for high oleic safflower and sunflower oils, produced from hybrid plants (if you can find them), which are structurally similar to olive oil, and, as a consequence, are more stable than traditional varieties).

Consistent with this last exception, canola oil is less problematical when heated, but there are some indications that canola oil presents dangers of its own. It goes rancid easier and develops mold quicker. Reports have shown that during the processing of canola oil, the omega-3 fatty acids are transformed into trans fatty acids. And, to top it all off, recent study indicates that canola oil can actually create deficiencies of vitamin E, the vitamin required for a healthy heart.

Flax seed oil is low in saturated fat and high in omega-3. As a result, flax seed oil provides a nice choice to correct the disproportionate amounts of omega-6/omega-3 fatty acids in the typical American diet. However, as noted in Part I, keep in mind that flaxseed oil has been linked to prostate cancer.

Palm and coconut oils are much more saturated than other vegetable oils. One of the main distinguishable benefits of coconut oil is that it has a special fatty acid, known as lauric acid, which can protect against bacteria and fungus. Historically, these oils have been used by countries in tropical climates. But, as these nations started to use more polyunsaturated vegetable oils, the incidence of intestinal disorders and immune deficiency diseases has increased demonstrably.

Palm and coconut oils are quite stable and can be kept at room temperature for many months without becoming rancid. These highly saturated tropical oils do not contribute to heart disease but have provided nourishment to healthy populations for a long, long time. They should be used more but they aren't due to the millions and millions of dollars of marketing expenditures (inclusive of lobbying efforts) by the vegetable oil industry in scaring people to avoid saturated fats.

So, what do you do in terms of consuming fats and oils? First, stay away from processed foods as they contain plenty of hydrogenated fats and polyunsaturated oils. Second, the vegetable oils you should use are olive oil, macadamia nut oil, sesame oil and to a limited degree unrefined expeller pressed flaxseed oil bottled in dark containers. Thirdly, consider cooking and baking with coconut oil. And, finally, don't hesitate to use butter, when it's desired, particularly good quality organic butter.

BUTTER OR MARGARINE

There has been a considerable amount of controversy surrounding butter versus margarine versus any other substitute spread. Studies on the potential cholesterol-raising effects of trans fatty acids have raised public concern about using margarine and whether other options, such as using butter (despite its high level of saturated fat and cholesterol), might be better choices. According to the American Heart Association, some stick margarines contribute more trans fatty acids than un-hydrogenated oils or other fats.

While studies have shown that using margarine can lower LDL ("bad") cholesterol when compared with butter, trans fatty acids in margarine can still raise LDL and lower HDL ("good") cholesterol.

Many so-called "experts" would seem to conclude that butter, being rich in both saturated fat and cholesterol, is potentially highly *"atherogenic"*, meaning it contributes to the build up of cholesterol and other substances in artery walls. However, it is not the butter that causes this, and the research is scant that butter and saturated fats cause chronic high cholesterol that is bad for you.[28]

Most margarine is made from vegetable fat and usually has (and marketed as containing) no dietary cholesterol. However, as more fully described in Chapter 8, cholesterol is not really your enemy. And, as described above (with respect to how fats are processed) the fact that margarine may be minimally hydrogenated or not hydrogenated at all still begs the question of its healthfulness or lack of it. Margarine, by virtue of the manner in which it is processed, has been linked to heart disease and cancer. The soft margarines or tub spreads, while lower in hydrogenated fats, are still produced from rancid vegetable oils and contain many additives.

I would unequivocally stay away from margarine. However, if you have to have margarine, the more liquid the margarine (in tub or liquid form), the less hydrogenated it is and the less trans fatty acids it contains. On the basis of current data, it is recommended that you should use naturally occurring, un-hydrogenated oil when possible.

The bottom line is that you need to really minimize, and ideally eliminate, your trans fat intake. If you limit your daily intake of fats and oils to 5-8 teaspoons, you aren't likely to get an excess of trans fatty acids. As noted above, the Food and Drug Administration (FDA) is requiring that food manufacturers list trans fat on food labels so it will be easier for consumers to avoid trans fats. As noted above, manufacturers have until January 1, 2006 to comply.

IF YOU HAVE CHILDREN TAKE HEED

As indicated *ad nauseum*, trans fats increase the risk for heart disease. But, children who start at age 3 or 4 eating a steady diet of fast food, pop tarts, commercially prepared fish sticks, stick margarine, cake, candy, cookies and microwave popcorn can be expected to get heart disease earlier than kids who are eating foods without trans fats.

While a person may not get heart disease until they are in their 40s, research at the University of Maryland has shown that kids as young as 8, 9 and 10 already have the high cholesterol and blood fats that clog arteries. By starting healthy eating habits early, parents can help their children avoid heart attacks and stroke.

What Steps Can Parents Take

Model healthy eating behaviors, make healthy choices available.

Try new fruits, vegetables, beans, chicken and other foods and recipes. Cook or prepare food more often as a family. Guard against fatigue because a tired parent can rely too heavily on fast foods or highly processed foods.

Learn how to identify high fat and trans fat foods.

When foods have a label, review the ingredient listing. Avoid foods labeled "hydrogenated or partially hydrogenated canola, soybean or cottonseed oil." The listing order for hydrogenated fats is important; if it is listed first, second, or third, there is a lot of it in the food. Foods that come from nature won't have trans or hydrogenated fats. Naturally low fat foods are generally the best: fruits of all types, vegetables, chicken, turkey, fish, beans, whole grains, breads and some cereals. These foods can be fixed in fun ways that your children will enjoy.

Learn the categories of foods that are likely to have trans fats

Some of the more common sources of trans fats are fast foods (like fried chicken, biscuits, fried fish sandwiches, French fries, fried apple or other pie desserts), donuts, muffins, crackers and most cookies, cake, cake icing, pie, pop tarts, microwave popped corn, canned biscuits, and meat pot pies.

Outsmart the profiteers who want you to be addicted to trans fats

Don't shop when you're hungry because you're more likely to make poor choices and buy on impulse when you shop on an empty stomach. If you take the children with you, give them a satisfying snack before you go. Stand firm in your plans about what you will and will not purchase.

Shop the perimeter of the store. Most of the processed foods, which contain a lot of trans fats, are on the inner isles of the supermarket. Have a plan for quick meals, snacks and lunch items you plan to purchase. Buy foods that you can fix quickly at home such as stir-fry packages, brown rice or couscous, chicken and wild salmon you can grill. And, when you do purchase processed foods, choose the lower fat versions of crackers, cereals and desserts.

Finally, remember that you are responsible for the quality of the foods you bring into the house for your children. Children eat the foods that are available to them.

AVOIDING TRANS FATS WHILE EATING OUT

In the supermarket, it's getting easier for you to avoid trans fat. Just read the labels.

And soon it should get even easier to avoid trans fat. As noted above, the Food and Drug Administration will require (in 2006) that trans fat levels be listed on all food labels. So, you'll be able to limit trans and saturated fats not just in margarines, but in shortening, cookies, cakes, frostings, doughnuts, pies, French fries, fried chicken, fried fish, and dozens of other foods.

The problem is that a good chunk of what we eat doesn't come with labels. One-third of all calories are now eaten outside your home – in restaurants, cafeterias, convenience stores, snack bars, and, especially, fast-food outlets. And, some of those foods make the trans levels in the supermarket aisles look trivial.

Despite the fact that some restaurant suppliers actually have direct replacements for the hydrogenated oil for use in most restaurants, for frying, most restaurants typically succumb to the pressure of profits, taste and cost cutting measures at the expense of the health of their customers. Here's a guide to dodging the trans fat that restaurants throw at you. The less you eat, the better.

Restaurant Rule # 1 – Cut Down on the Appetizers.

Eliminate most of the appetizers. Remember when an appetizer meant shrimp cocktail, consommé, or other light fare to whet your appetite? Now, today's appetizers are more likely to crush the ones just mentioned, and your chances of not moving up a size by next swimsuit season. Take the ever-popular batter-dipped fried whole onion plus dipping sauce that's served at steak houses. It's not just an appetizer – it's a day's worth of calories (2,100) and trans fat (18 grams). Add in its saturated fat and you're talking about a four-day supply of arterial sludge.

Those delectable cheese fries with ranch dressing at many restaurants are another marvel of modern face stuffing. Their 11 grams of trans fat are bad enough. Add 81 grams of saturated fat at the same time along with the 3000 calories that they have and you are just plain accelerating your heart disease.

And so it goes. From stuffed potato skins to fried mozzarella sticks to buffalo wings, the typical appetizer menu brings good business to fat farms and funeral parlors. Whether it starts out fatty (like the cheese sticks and chicken wings) or ends up that way (what with frying and dipping sauce), you end up with a huge amount of trans (plus saturated) fat and calories.

Restaurant Rule # 2 – Develop a Fear of Frying.

At home, it's fine to sauté in a little canola or olive oil (or even better from the standpoint of reduced free radical activity – macadamia nut oil or coconut oil). At fast food and mid-priced restaurants, many foods are fried in what starts out as a brick or sludge-like shortening or margarine. And that means a sizeable dose of trans fat.

Seafood restaurants are a good example. A typical order of fried clams or the fried seafood combo packs about 50 grams of fat, roughly ten of them trans fat and almost as many saturated. At seafood chains the fried shrimp, fried fish, and fried everything else mean heart trouble.

Dinner-house and family-style chains apparently buy their shortening from the same distributors as seafood restaurants judging by the six to ten grams of trans fat in each order of onion rings or chicken fingers. The same is the case for fast-food chains. One company's fried chicken dinner has seven grams of trans fat, mostly from the chicken and biscuit.

Of course, one restaurant food probably delivers more trans fat to the nation's circulatory system than any other – French fries. These artery clogging deep fried potato sticks are sold just about everywhere but your local coffee shop or bookstore. The most popular side dish in America (at the major fast food chains) provides anywhere from four grams to seven grams of trans fat to the arteries. Even if the chains use liquid oil in the restaurants, they rely on hydrogenated fats to prefry the fries <u>before</u> shipping.

Restaurant Rule # 3 – Don't Focus Just on Hydrogenated Oils.

Not all trans fat comes from hydrogenated vegetable oil. Meat and milk have small amounts of naturally occurring trans fat. But "small" becomes substantial (seven grams) when you're ordering a 16-ounce prime rib. A chicken pot pie has six grams of trans (and 11 grams of saturated fat) lurking in that innocent – looking pastry dough. And, are you looking forward to that nice "hearty" (the ultimate misnomer) breakfast of biscuits and gravy. That will start your day with four grams of trans fat (plus ten grams of saturated fat).

Restaurant Rule # 4 – Be Real Careful of Pastries

The term "pastries" is quite interesting. The purveyors of many other unhealthy foods have created a façade of benefits and attractiveness designed to titillate your taste buds and cause you to devour the food at your first chance. They even have names for them that sound tempting and delicious, like "cookies", "candies", "burgers", "fries" and so forth. However, with "pastries", there is no such pulling of the punches. In fact, the marketers are telling you right off the bat that the food is made of an artery clogging "paste." Remember when you mixed water and flour in kindergarten. Pastries are simply loaded with a bunch of saturated and trans fats. It is just a matter of how much. One simple case in point – it is fascinating that one can devour a cinnamon bun at one major chain with 670 calories and 34 grams of fat!

Restaurant Rule # 5 – Try to Reduce Your Salt Intake

Table salt might very well be one of the most deadly ingredients in the food supply. Salt is one of the major causes of high blood pressure in the U.S., which increases risks of heart attack, congestive heart failure, stroke and kidney disease.

The salt in our diets has turned our hearts and arteries into ticking time bombs that explode in tens of thousands of Americans every year in terms of causing high blood pressure. Our country has become addicted to salt because once again manufacturers and restaurants use more of it because it makes food taste good and if it tastes good people will buy it. And, if more people buy it the restaurant and/or the manufacturer will make more money. This vicious cycle cannot be stopped without legislative intervention because if one manufacturer or restaurant stops or reduces salt in foods they prepare or create, their competitor will not and, once again, it just does not make good business sense. The bottom line is trading off the profits of business for consumers' health.

So much has been focused on calories, carbs and fats over the years, salt has been forgotten, particularly with overwhelming and excessive use of blood pressure drugs. After all, the American consumer can "enjoy" his or her food and if it causes high blood pressure, just pop a pill. Again, as long as there is no pain involved, everything is all right. Americans will get more concerned over the taste of a certain food they are eating than the consequences and side effects of the drugs that they take. Salt consumption has steadily increased in the last several decades, with Americans consuming a daily average of 3,375 milligrams of sodium, over 50% more than the amount recommended by the federal government, which is roughly a teaspoon.

A glaring example of this is a typical top brand turkey frozen dinner having 5,410 milligrams just by itself. Another example is well known breakfast on the menu at a national restaurant chain – 4,462 milligrams of sodium.

The natural salt content in food accounts for just 10 percent of total salt intake, while discretionary salt use accounts for 5 percent or 10 percent more. The remainder comes from salt added by manufacturers, making it difficult for Americans to eat a low-sodium diet.

Restaurant Rule #6 – Order to Avoid the Harmful Trans Fats

On the positive side, plenty of restaurant fare is nearly trans fat free. Your best bet is to order food that's low in all fats. For example, at most delis, get the turkey sandwich with mustard. At seafood restaurants, order broiled fish. If you are stuck at a dinner-house chain, try the barbecue or grilled chicken breast. At fast food places, order a grilled chicken deluxe sandwich without the mayo. Pick lower-fat Chinese dishes like szechuan shrimp or stir-fried vegetables. It's a good bet that the cook is using liquid oil. And if you steer clear of the beef, pork, and deep-fried ingredients, you will not get a heavy dose of omega-6 fatty acids. Most salads should also be low in trans fat. But, the dressing with its high polyunsaturated and even trans fat content will be defeating your purposes, not to mention the omega-6 fatty acids from any meat that you use.

THE ADDED CARCINOGENIC RISKS OF CERTAIN TARGETED FOODS AND FOOD PREPARATION

Given all that has been discussed about the cardiovascular risks of saturated fats and trans fats, one thing that is often overlooked is the consequences of free radical and carcinogenic activity as a result of preparing and cooking certain foods. You learned above about hydrogenation and the creation of free radicals from the extraction with respect to certain oils and how excessive heat (from frying, for example) can create free radicals.

Another discovery involves a cancer-causing chemical in certain fried and baked starchy foods. For example, popular American brands of snack chips and French fries contain disturbingly high levels of acrylamide (which is sometimes used in water treatment facilities), according to laboratory tests commissioned by the Center for Science in the Public Interest (CSPI) in 2005. Acrylamide forms as a result of unknown chemical reactions during high-temperature baking or frying. The tests were conducted by the same Swedish government scientists that two months earlier had discovered that several popular brands of snack chips, taco shells, French fries, and breakfast cereals were shown to have some of the highest acrylamide levels.

Fast-food French fries showed the highest levels of acrylamide among the foods tested, with large orders containing 39 to 72 micrograms. One-ounce portions of famous brand potato crisps contained about 25 micrograms, with other corn-based products containing half that amount or less. A notable brand of breakfast cereals contained 6 or 7 micrograms of the carcinogenic substance. The amount of acrylamide in a large order of fast-food French fries is at least 300 times more than what the U.S. Environmental Protection Agency allows in a glass of water.

EVEN OUR COURT SYSTEM IS GETTING ON THE BANDWAGON

On February 12, 2005, McDonald's agreed to pay $8.5 million to settle a lawsuit over artery-clogging trans fats in its cooking oils. McDonald's agreed to donate $7 million to the American Heart Association and spend another $1.5 million to inform the public of its trans fat plans.

The settlement was the result of litigation from a San Francisco area activist who has been seeking to raise public awareness of the health dangers from the trans fatty acids in hydrogenated or partially hydrogenated oils. Stephen Joseph, a lawyer who founded *bantransfats.com*, sued McDonald's over complaints the firm did not properly inform the public that it had encountered delays in plans to lessen the trans fats in its cooking oils. Joseph first gained publicity for his cause by suing Kraft Foods in 2003 to highlight the trans fat content of much-beloved Oreo cookies. The company has since moved to remove trans fats from its snack foods.

It is sad that it had to get to the point of suing this country's largest corporations to force them to stop sacrificing the health of Americans for their own greed. Again, this continues to illustrate that we must be proactive in deciding what constitutes healthy food and what constitutes dangerous foodstuffs imposed upon unsuspecting and uneducated consumers by profiteering multi-billion dollar corporations.

In early 2005, a California attorney formally demanded that McDonald's and Burger King place a cancer warning on their French fries, as required by the state's Proposition 65. Burger King faced a legal deadline of late June and McDonald's of that year to respond.

PARTING THOUGHTS ON FATS

Your management of the fats you consume is one of the smartest things you can do for not only your heart health, but for your overall well-being. Let's review some of the practical tips that I went over in this chapter that you can use every day to keep your consumption of problematical fats under control while consuming a nutritionally adequate diet.

First, check the Nutrition Facts panel to compare foods because the serving sizes are generally consistent in similar types of foods. Choose foods lower in saturated fat and cholesterol, but particularly trans fat. For saturated fat and cholesterol, keep in mind that 5 percent of the daily value or less is low and 20 percent or more is high.

Second, choose your fats wisely. Do not categorically replace saturated fats in your diet with polyunsaturated fats. Many polyunsaturated fats (the way they are now manufactured) are worse overall than saturated fats. There are many hidden dangers in polyunsaturated fats that have been overlooked by many. Saturated fats, such as macadamia nut oil and sesame oil that do not become unstable under heated cooking conditions are also good. Sources of monounsaturated fats such as olive oil are a wise choice to eat unheated. Get your good polyunsaturated fats from fish (when eaten in moderation), nuts and flaxseed and avoid soybean, corn and sunflower oils.

Third, stay away from shortenings and hard margarines. You may choose vegetable oils and soft margarines (liquid, tub, or spray) because you may believe the amounts of saturated fat, trans fat, and cholesterol are lower than the amounts in saturated vegetable oils such as coconut and palm oils, and animal fats, including butter. But, that belief is not warranted, in my view. Many saturated fats are good for you as described above in this chapter.

However, if that is your choice, consider beefing up on fruits, vegetables and antioxidants, since these vegetable oils and soft margarines generate a significant amount of free radicals when cooked. Using vegetable oils and soft margarine has the effect of increasing your cancer risk and otherwise damaging many of your bodily processes. Unfortunately, free radicals are actually byproducts of our bodies' normal metabolic process and these compounds interfere with the ability of certain cells to function normally. They attack and weaken cells and tissues and contribute to disease, and antioxidants (inclusive of fruits and vegetables) help to stop them.

If buying and preparing an adequate amount of raw fruits and vegetables is a problem, a good source of fruits and vegetables is a product known as JuicePlus+, which contains 5-6 servings of fruits and vegetables in pill form (see www.juiceplus. com/+sk27973). Since the recent guidelines for daily recommended intake of fruits and vegetables has increased to 5-13 servings per day, these pills provide a good base and all additional servings of actual food should be right within the optimum amount.

Fourth, choose lean meats, such as poultry (remember not to eat the skin) and bison (buffalo). Don't fry your meats and trim off the visible fat.

Fifth, ask before you order when eating out. A good tip to remember is to ask which fats are being used in the preparation of your food when eating or ordering out. Don't be shy in asking your waitperson to eliminate salt or reduce the salt, or any seasoning to which you may be sensitive. I am sensitive to garlic, sad to say, so I am always on guard and proactive in that respect.

Sixth, watch your calories, as fats are high in calories. All sources of fat contain nine calories per gram, making fat the most concentrated source of calories. By comparison, carbohydrates and protein have only four calories per gram.

Chapter 8
Lower Your Cholesterol and Your Drugs Without Lowering Your Standards – Naturally

"Give a man a fish and you feed him for a day. Teach a man to fish and you feed him for a lifetime."

—Chinese Proverb

A discussion of cardiovascular issues would not be complete without dealing with the issue of cholesterol. But, has cholesterol gotten a bad rap? Is "low" or the "lowest possible" cholesterol something that you really want to achieve? Can your cholesterol actually be too low? And, what is the meaning and real impact of the notions of "good" and "bad" cholesterol?

Chapter 8 will focus on what cholesterol is really all about. I will analyze how bad (LDL) cholesterol becomes "bad" in the first place (in reality, LDL is actually supposed to do positive things for your body). I will also discuss what are the optimum cholesterol levels. And, I will focus on why there is such a predominance of, and reliance upon, prescription drugs as a quick fix to one of America's most exaggerated health problems. The last section of this chapter will suggest some natural supplements and lifestyle changes that should help with any cholesterol problems that you may have.

YOU NEED YOUR CHOLESTEROL

To begin with, me explain what cholesterol is and what it does in your body. Cholesterol is produced naturally in your liver and it helps with important body functions.

Along with saturated fats, cholesterol gives your cells necessary stiffness and stability. Recall, if you will, our discussion of polyunsaturated fats in Chapter 7. Now, when your diet contains an excess of polyunsaturated fatty acids, these replace saturated fatty acids in your cell membrane, so that your cell walls actually become flabby. When this happens, cholesterol from your blood is "driven" from your blood into your tissues to give them structural integrity. This is why serum cholesterol levels may go down temporarily when you replace saturated fats with polyunsaturated oils in your diet.

Cholesterol leads to the development of vital hormones that help you deal with stress and protects your body against heart disease and cancer (these are called "*corticosteroids*") and certain of your sex hormones.

Dietary cholesterol plays an important role in maintaining the health of your intestines, which is why low-cholesterol vegetarian diets can lead to leaky gut syndrome and other intestinal disorders. Further, it also allows for better digestion of fats in your diet through the creation of bile salts.

Cholesterol is important in the creation of your very valuable vitamin D stores, which is critical if you want healthy bones and nervous system, proper growth, mineral metabolism, muscle tone, insulin production, reproduction and immune system function. Babies and children need cholesterol-rich foods throughout their growing years to ensure proper development of the brain and nervous system. If you are a nursing mother, your milk is particularly rich in cholesterol and contains a special enzyme that helps your baby utilize the cholesterol most efficiently.

And, probably as important as anything, cholesterol acts as an antioxidant. Most likely, this is why cholesterol levels go up with age.

THE CHEMICAL MAKE-UP OF YOUR CHOLESTEROL

Cholesterol is often called a "lipid" or fat. Its numerous carbon and hydrogen atoms are put together in an intricate three-dimensional network, impossible to dissolve in water. All living creatures use this "in-dissolvability" cleverly, incorporating cholesterol into their cell walls to make cells waterproof. This means that your cells can regulate your internal environment undisturbed by changes in your surroundings, a mechanism vital for the proper function of your body. The fact that your cells are waterproof is especially critical for the normal functioning of your nerves and nerve cells. Thus, the highest concentration of cholesterol in your body is found in your brain and other parts of your nervous system.

Because cholesterol is insoluble in water and thus also in your blood, it is transported in your blood inside spherical particles composed of fats (lipids) and proteins, the so-called lipoproteins. Your lipoproteins, on the other hand, are easily dissolved in water because their outside is composed mainly of water-soluble proteins. The inside of your lipoproteins is composed of lipids where there is room for water-insoluble molecules such as cholesterol. Lipoproteins are like taxis, carrying cholesterol from one place in the body to another.

THE TASKS OF YOUR LDLS AND YOUR HDLS

The lipoproteins have various names based upon their density. As I alluded to earlier in Chapter 7 on trans fats, the best known are HDL (high density lipoprotein), and LDL (low density lipoprotein). The main task of your HDL is to carry cholesterol from your peripheral tissues, including the artery walls, to your liver. Here, your HDL is excreted with your bile, or used for other purposes, for instance as a starting point for the manufacture of important hormones. Your LDL mainly transports cholesterol in the opposite direction. Cholesterol is carried from the liver, where most of your body's cholesterol is produced, to the peripheral tissues, including the vascular walls. When your cells need cholesterol, they call for the LDLs, which then deliver cholesterol into the interior of your cells. Did you know that most of the cholesterol in your blood, (between 60 and 80 per cent) is transported by LDL and is paradoxically called "bad" cholesterol? And, only 15-20 percent is transported by HDL and called "good" cholesterol. A small part of the circulating cholesterol is transported by other lipoproteins.

Contrary to popular belief, about 80% of your cholesterol does <u>not</u> come from the things that you eat. Rather, it is synthesized by your liver. A special enzyme (the name of which is too long and cumbersome to identify here) controls the formation of cholesterol (this formation process is more appropriately called "*biosynthesis*"). Dietary changes can merely influence your cholesterol levels. When cholesterol levels are low, liver production of the enzyme increases to speed biosynthesis of cholesterol. Conversely, when cholesterol levels are too high, the liver limits enzyme production to reduce cholesterol production. Proper functioning of this feedback mechanism is vital for the maintenance of healthy cholesterol levels.

LDLs, HDLs and Atherosclerosis

Surprisingly, atherosclerosis does not happen when your LDLs are doing its proper job. Unfortunately, modern dietary habits (such as excess intake of certain polyunsaturated fats, trans fatty acids and some saturated fats), genetic disorders and lifestyle contribute to the disruption of this system of your liver regulating cholesterol levels and LDLs delivering cholesterol to your blood vessels. These poor eating habits and lifestyle lead to elevated amounts of free radicals and cholesterol levels (and correlated LDL levels). When all of these are present at the same time, very bad things can happen in your body.

Let's say that you are an unhealthy person that is creating too many free radicals and has too much LDL in your blood. When LDL is directed to lesions in your endothelial cells (remember, they are that thin layer of flat cells that line your blood vessels as well as other cavities and vessels) lining the inner walls of blood vessels, deposits are formed in your arterial walls. The deposited LDL undergoes modification, as free radicals oxidize LDL to form special types of cells that create a thick, hard plaque.

Over time, plaque accumulation can constrict vessels, inhibiting blood flow and reducing the supply of oxygen reaching the heart, brain, and other organs. If a clot (thrombus) blocks an artery already restricted by plaque, blood and oxygen flow can be cut off entirely, leading to a heart attack (if the occlusion occurs in the heart) or a stroke (if it occurs in the brain).

HDL helps remove excess cholesterol from atherosclerotic deposits that you may have and retard the growth of new plaque. If you have low HDL levels, you will be at higher mortality risk from coronary artery disease and strokes, particularly if you are elderly.

Taking LDLs to the Next Level – A Marker that is Sometimes Overlooked

To take the above discussion one step further, in order to bind with other molecules for transport through your circulatory system, lipids rely on a specialized class of structural proteins, called *apoproteins*. LDL actually exists in two versions. The first is called "*apolipoprotein A*", and consists of a large, "fluffy" protein called *apoprotein A* that is cardioprotective when bound to LDL. The second, called *"apolipoprotein B"*, consists of a small, dense protein called *apoprotein B* that plays a major role in cardiovascular disease when bound to LDL. Apolipoprotein-B particles enable cholesterol to penetrate and lodge in vascular walls, an important step in initiating the formation of atherosclerotic plaque. Apolipoprotein B is the predominant form of apolipoprotein, and over 90% of all LDL cholesterol particles in the blood carry apolipoprotein B, making it an especially accurate (and convenient) marker for measuring the cholesterol-depositing capacity of blood.

WHY "HIGH" CHOLESTEROL IS OVERRATED

The focus on cholesterol as being the culprit is actually effective for one thing – selling over-priced drugs and shock value panic. The real truth lies deeper than simply saying that cholesterol needs to be low and that you need expensive drugs to get it there. It is submitted that the "high cholesterol" craze is a shallow money-making myth manufactured by the drug companies.

Actually, the plaque in your arteries isn't made up of naturally occurring cholesterol. It is made up of a special kind of cholesterol, which is "oxidized" cholesterol caused by free radical damage. Again, the marketers for the drug companies have "framed" cholesterol for the "rap" that was caused by other reasons because it has been financially beneficial to do so. In essence, cholesterol really isn't that bad. Moreover, cholesterol is not a deadly poison, but a substance vital to your cells.

Your blood vessels can become damaged in a number of ways-through irritations caused by free radicals or viruses, or because they are structurally weak. When this happens, cholesterol, as your body's natural healing substance, steps in to repair the damage. In addition, your cholesterol itself may be damaged by exposure to heat and oxygen, which usually occurs from frying your foods and cooking them through other high-temperature processes. This damaged or oxidized cholesterol can potentially cause injury to, and a buildup of plaque in, your arteries.

If you have high serum cholesterol levels, this usually indicates that your body needs cholesterol to protect itself from high levels of the altered, free radical-containing fats. In short, cholesterol is needed if your body is poorly nourished to protect you from heart disease and cancer.

If you are under mental stress, undergo physical activity or change your body weight, you may influence the level of your blood cholesterol. High cholesterol is not dangerous by itself, but may reflect an unhealthy condition, or it may be totally innocent. The term "high cholesterol" is often viewed as being bad when, in reality, it is intended to mean that you have too much "bad" LDL cholesterol in your system. Also, having too much "bad" cholesterol is more of a marker of heart disease rather than a cause.

If you have gray hair society might view you as getting older. But, did the gray hair cause you to get old? If you dyed your hair to reduce the gray would if really make you any younger? Hardly. The same is true with your cholesterol. Maybe something else is causing both the gray hair and aging. Similarly, even if cholesterol is elevated, maybe something else is causing the elevated cholesterol and something else is also causing the heart disease.

One of the main reasons why cholesterol has been blamed for so much of the heart health problems is that the big business marketers and food suppliers have presupposed that you and most Americans are unhealthy eaters and have unhealthy lifestyles. And, as explained throughout this Part II, it is these same big business marketers and food suppliers that overload our food stores and restaurants with unhealthy non-nutritious foods for you to eat. Thus, if it is presumed that you and virtually everyone else eat unhealthfully, it necessarily follows that you will have problematical high serum cholesterol levels. Again, this is because your body needs cholesterol to protect itself from high levels of the chemically altered and free radical-containing foods that promote free radical activity in your body. And, it is this free radical activity, which turns cholesterol from something good for you to something bad for you. Cholesterol has gotten the bad rap because it is beautifully convenient and profitable from a marketing standpoint – plain and simple.

Why Good and Why Bad

You may ask why cholesterol, which is a natural substance in your blood with important biologic functions, is called "bad" when it is transported from the liver to the rest of your body by LDL, but called "good" when HDL transports it the other way? The reason is that a number of studies have shown that a lower-than-normal level of HDL-cholesterol and a higher than-normal level of LDL-cholesterol are associated with a greater risk of having a heart attack. Conversely, a higher-than-normal level of HDL-cholesterol and a lower-than normal LDL-cholesterol is associated with a smaller risk. Or, said in another way, a low HDL/LDL ratio is a risk factor for coronary heart disease.

However, as noted above, a risk factor is not necessarily the same as the cause. Something may provoke a heart attack and at the same time lower the HDL/LDL ratio. Many factors are known to influence this ratio.

Let's say that you reduce your body weight. Well, you will also reduce your cholesterol. Interestingly, only cholesterol transported by LDL goes down; the small part transported by HDL goes up. In other words, your weight reduction increases the ratio between HDL and LDL cholesterol. An increase of the HDL/LDL ratio is considered to be "favorable" by the diet-heart supporters. But is the ratio or the weight reduction the measurement that is favorable? When you become fat, other harmful things occur to you. One is that your cells become less sensitive to insulin, so that you can develop diabetes. And, if you have diabetes you are much more likely to have a heart attack than people without diabetes, because atherosclerosis and other vascular damage occur very early in diabetics (even if you don't have cholesterol problems). In other words, being overweight may increase the risk of a heart attack by mechanisms other than unfavorable cholesterol levels, while at the same time being overweight lowers the HDL/LDL ratio.

Also, if you are a smoker, cholesterol will increase to a degree. Again, it is your LDL-cholesterol that increases, while your HDL-cholesterol drops, resulting in an "unfavorable" HDL/LDL ratio. However, what is really unfavorable is the chronic exposure to the fumes from burning paper and tobacco leaves. Instead of considering the low HDL/LDL ratio as bad it could simply be smoking itself that is bad. Smoking may provoke a heart attack and, *at the same time*, lower the HDL/LDL ratio.

A low ratio is also associated with high blood pressure. Most probably, the hypertensive effect is created by your sympathetic nervous system, which is often over-stimulated if you have high blood pressure. Hypertension or too much adrenalin may provoke a heart attack by inducing a spasm of the coronary arteries or by stimulating the arterial muscle cells to proliferate, and, at the same time, lower the HDL/LDL ratio.

As you see, knowing what is bad is not easy. Is it bad for you to be fat, to smoke, to be inactive, to have high blood pressure, or to be stressed? Or is it bad for you to have a lot of bad cholesterol – or both? Is it good for you to be slim, to stop smoking, to exercise, to have normal blood pressure, to be emotionally calm? Or is it good for you to have much "good" cholesterol – or both? Thus, the chance of you having a heart attack is greater than normal if you have high LDL cholesterol, but so is the risk if you are fat, sedentary, a smoker, hypertensive and mentally stressed. And, if you have elevated levels of LDL cholesterol, it is, of course, impossible to know whether the increased risk is due to the previously mentioned risk factors (or to other risk factors that are presently unknown) or to the high LDL cholesterol. To ignore these other risk factors (the ones other than high LDL cholesterol) would seem to make the analysis of heart health somewhat meaningless. To prove that high LDL cholesterol is an independent risk factor, we should inquire if fat, sedentary, smoking, hypertensive and mentally stressed individuals with a high LDL cholesterol level are at greater risk for coronary disease than fat, sedentary, smoking, hypertensive and mentally stressed individuals with low or normal LDL cholesterol.

CHOLESTEROL LOWERING STATIN DRUGS – A DEVIL IN DISGUISE

Cholesterol lowering drugs (or "statin" drugs as they are called in the trade) are extremely popular in America. They bring to the drug companies over $20 billion per year in the United States (this was as of the end of 2004)! And, the situation continues to become even scarier as these companies continue to influence the manipulation of (by lowering) national cholesterol guidelines to bring a whole new meaning to their drugs on a national scale. And, they further promote that you need to adopt a low fat diet to lower cholesterol.

The sad truth, however, is that the drug companies know that mainstream America cannot adopt a correct (not necessarily low fat) diet for a variety of reasons – cost, taste, accessibility just to name a few. Moreover, it is simply not profitable to have a food distribution system that universally provides organic fruits and vegetables, and much lower unhealthy fats and sugary carbohydrates. The financial paradox is that if these so-called healthy foods predominated the shelves of our food stores and the menus of our restaurants, then you and most everyone else would become less of a consumer of the food products that are provided by the purveyors of such foodstuffs. This is mainly because you would necessarily be getting the nutrition you need – and you would spend less. If unhealthy, fat-laden, high carb foods, continue to dominate like they do now, then you will continue to crave these foods – you will continue to devour pleasant tasting sauces, delightfully aromatic and palate-soothing fried foods, "creamy" dairy products, foods infused with sweet sugars of all varieties, flavorful salts, and not to mention yummy pastries and gastronomical cakes. They taste good, they are cheaper and you and people all over the world keep coming back for more. However, ironically, as the human body continues to cry out for nutrition, it is fed more and more of the things that do just the opposite.

You, like most other consumers, have been led like sheep to focus on taste, as food suppliers have been led to focus on profits. And, what do you get in reality? Well, you wind up with fatty sauces, artery-clogging, carcinogenic fried foods, blood pressure spiking salts, trans fat laden pastries and cakes and sugars that cause or promote high insulin levels (which can lead to high blood pressure), high cholesterol, heart disease, diabetes, weight gain, premature aging, suppression of the immune system, weakened defenses against bacterial infection, hyperactivity and attention deficit disorder in children and many more negative side effects. These foods have minimal nutritional value and otherwise wreak havoc on the efficient operation of our bodily processes. And, you wonder why our healthcare system is overburdened!

Be that as it may, our drug companies have continued the hypocrisy by providing us with another convenience – low cholesterol in a pill. If you cannot, or don't have the will to, prevent it, simply pop it! People in this country and even world-wide have been led to believe that they need to take expensive "statin" prescription drugs in pill form to prevent them from having a condition that they believe will cause them to fall prey to the number one killer in the United States, notably heart disease. Guidelines heavily lobbied for by the drug companies have now caused approximately a whopping 36 million Americans to qualify for these prescription drugs!

Do they lower cholesterol? Yes, they do. Statins lower cholesterol levels by inhibiting the production of that enzyme (discussed above which synthesizes cholesterol in the liver), resulting in a decrease in cholesterol synthesis. To compensate for the resulting reduction of cholesterol production, the liver begins to remove LDL circulating in the blood, further reducing overall LDL levels. But, remember, LDLs are not inherently (by themselves) bad for you, as they serve a useful bodily function.

Statins are supposedly tremendously effective and they are claimed to be completely safe at the recommended dosages. Unfortunately, the statins' success in lowering cholesterol has led many people to believe they represent a cure-all for cholesterol and heart disease risk. They are not, however, a cure-all. And, what about the side effects of these drugs? Studies have shown that 98 per cent of patients taking Lipitor developed muscle pain and/or weakness, and one third of those on Mevacor developed the problem.

What physicians, who prescribe these drugs, often overlook is that patients taking them become depleted in our good friend, coenzyme Q10 (CoQ10), which I discussed in detail in Chapter 5. This can lead to fatigue, muscle weakness, soreness and heart failure in and of itself.

If you start with relatively low CoQ10 levels (the elderly and patients with heart failure) begin to manifest signs/symptoms of CoQ10 deficiency relatively rapidly – in six to 12 months. Younger patients, however, can tolerate the statins for several years before they begin developing symptoms.

Now muscle problems would be bad enough, especially if they prevent you from, for example, putting your foot on the brake when you need to while driving. But statins also have been shown to cause cancer, neuropathy (nerve damage), dizziness, memory failure, and depression. These drugs are even known to cause heart failure itself.

Lovastin, a commonly prescribed drug for lowering blood cholesterol, sold by Merck and Co. under the name *Mevacor*, may affect people's ability to drive or perform other everyday tasks. In other words, *Lovastatin* could affect attention and reaction speed. Studies have shown that patients who had been given *Lovastatin* showed decreased attention and psychomotor speed, compared with those who had not received the drug. Those who had the greatest decreases in cholesterol levels suffered the greatest impairment.

The Bottom Line on Cholesterol-Lowering Prescription Drugs

Being that the cardio-protective benefits of statin drugs are viewed by most as outweighing the known side effects, it appears that tens of millions of new patients will be taking statins for a period of decades, and possibly for a lifetime. Unfortunately, data on the long-term use of statins is scant. But, what about the possibility of long-term statin use causing cancer? There have been studies that suggest this. While conceding that this is an uncertain process, it is submitted that consideration be made to avoid statins except in cases where there is a short-term risk of coronary heart disease, and consider more natural strategies discussed in the *Natural Cholesterol Solution I – What You Should Do,* discussed in the next several pages of this chapter.

There is no argument that statin prescription drugs work, but they simply do not treat the cause of the problem. These drugs are potentially dangerous to your health and are really nothing more than an expensive, potentially toxic "band-aid" approach to curing, instigated by the ulterior agendas of profiteering multi-billion dollar drug companies. These drugs simply do not address the cause of the problem, and consequently, the underlying condition that is causing the risk factor (high cholesterol) will crop up and eventually cause other diseases.

Simply stated, statin drugs are not the only way to lower your cholesterol if your cholesterol is high, let alone high cholesterol not being that bad in the first place (assuming that cholesterol is not excessively high as noted in the previous section).

HOW LOW IS TOO LOW

Most people are worried about having cholesterol levels that are too high, yet there are studies which reveal that low cholesterol is actually associated with adverse bodily functions and behavioral effects.

While the medical establishment continues to push the suppression of cholesterol levels to abnormally low levels, it is not widely known that there is a significant amount of evidence linking low cholesterol to aggressive behavior and depression according to researchers from Yale University School of Medicine. This is due to cholesterol's role in developing serotonin, the "feel good" hormone that regulates mood.

Low levels of cholesterol in the blood may also increase stroke risk. The study linking low cholesterol to increased stroke risk was presented recently at the 24th American Heart Association Conference on Stroke and Cerebral Circulation. Low cholesterol levels have been shown to worsen individuals that have congestive heart failure, that life-threatening condition where the heart becomes too weak to effectively pump blood. Statin drugs have been shown to also cause nerve damage and to greatly impair memory. A reason for statin drugs having these various serious side effects is that they work by slowing up a vital enzyme that manufactures cholesterol in your liver. However, that same enzyme is used to manufacture CoQ10 (that chemical in your body that is needed to transfer energy from food to your cells to be used for keeping you alive and staying healthy).

Low cholesterol is necessary to maintain integrity of the vessel wall. Very low levels of cholesterol, however, might lead to "leaky vessels." The Japanese have typically low cholesterol levels and a higher than average rate of hemorrhagic stroke.

Frankly, the optimum cholesterol is about 200, contrary to popular belief. Levels below 180 appear to be a problem, with levels under 150 are a major serious problem.

THE NATURAL CHOLESTEROL SOLUTION I – WHAT YOU SHOULD DO

There are some natural and safe protocols and supplements that not only lower cholesterol, but also provide a host of other benefits. Sound familiar and repetitive? Well, I intended it to be.

The very basic mandate in a very general sense is to have a diet low in some saturated and polyunsaturated fats and high in fruits and vegetables. Beyond that there is a whole host of specific supplements (which I will describe below) that have shown positive benefits in terms of preventative and restorative heart health. For preventative maintenance, the dosages on the bottles are fairly good evidence of the proper dosage. However, for therapeutic doses, consult a professional who has considerable experience in nutritional supplementation, and this does not necessarily mean a medical doctor. Most physicians won't know any more than you do about the supplements mentioned in this book, particularly after you are done reading it. So, consider consulting with a naturopathic or osteopathic physician, or even a chiropractor. If you are currently under cardiac care, advise your doctor that you plan to add supplements to your diet.

The following are my suggestions to afford you opportunity to normalize your cholesterol levels.

Fruits, Vegetables and Antioxidants

More Fruits and Vegetables

A diet rich in fiber and vegetables works just as well at controlling your increased cholesterol levels. Pectin, found in apples and the rinds of citrus fruits, is a natural fiber that lowers cholesterol; these same foods also provide flavonoids that yield broad health-promoting effects.

Flavonoids

A large and diverse collection of naturally occurring substances that lower cholesterol, flavonoids provide antioxidant benefits, lower blood pressure, possess anti-inflammatory properties, and prevent cancer.[29] There is a product distributed by the Life Extension Foundation called Sytrinol™, which is a new, patented complex of citrus bioflavonoid. It is a convenient way to lower LDL by as much as 15% while obtaining all the other benefits of flavonoids. However, in one test conducted using this product containing these substances, the subjects saw reductions of 30% in total cholesterol, 27% in LDL, and 34% in total triglycerides! In addition, HDL levels increased 4%, resulting in a significant 29% reduction in the LDL/HDL ratio.

Antioxidants

Vitamins

I noted previously in this chapter that cholesterol itself is not bad but oxidized cholesterol, ravaged by free radicals is bad. The best way to protect against free radical damage is by supplying your body with antioxidants. Vitamin C and E are known to be the best, safest antioxidants to protect against heart disease and this has been confirmed by many studies. Actually, high levels of vitamin C can protect the level of vitamin E (ideally in the form of tocotrienols) in your tissues.

Vitamin C is excellent at lessening the risk of stroke and heart attacks, strengthening blood vessels, and reducing blood pressure, fibrinogen levels, inflammation and C-reactive protein. Vitamin E prevents plaque formation, protects LDL from oxidation, strengthens blood vessels, reduces blood pressure, reduces blood viscosity and platelet aggregation, reduces C-reactive protein, and is helpful in atrial fibrillation and ventricular fibrillation.

Minerals

A review published in the October 2004 issue of the *Journal of the American College of Nutrition* has found that many cardiovascular benefits of magnesium parallel those of statin drugs (the class of drugs commonly prescribed for individuals with elevated cholesterol levels, a traditional risk factor for cardiovascular disease noted above).

The researchers discussed the fact that both statin drugs and magnesium can inactivate the enzyme responsible for the first step in cholesterol formation and improve the function of blood vessels, reduce inflammation, and provide other cardiovascular benefits. Magnesium, however, is also involved in the activity of another enzyme known as "*LCAT*", which helps elevate beneficial HDL cholesterol levels while reducing unhealthy LDL cholesterol and triglycerides. In addition, magnesium is necessary for the enzyme that converts linoleic acid and linolenic acid into compounds that reduce inflammation. Furthermore, as you will learn in Chapter 10, optimal levels of magnesium within the cell are a natural calcium channel blocker, which helps dilate the blood vessels.

The "bottom line" is that magnesium has many cardiovascular benefits, is relatively low cost, and has a good safety profile. What more could you ask for!

Other Antioxidants

There is one antioxidant that even mainstream medical doctors are claiming can dramatically improve the action of other antioxidants, such as vitamin C and E, coenzyme Q10 and glutathione. It is alpha-lipoic acid (ALA), which is one of the best antioxidants you can take.[30] Unlike vitamins C and E, which only work in water and fat respectively, ALA overpowers free radicals in both fat and water. Plus, as vitamins C and E subdue free radicals, they lose electrons. But ALA actually helps restore those lost electrons so C and E can go on fighting!

ALA is produced naturally by your body but as you age, your body produces less and less ALA so, supplementing is necessary. Plus, in addition to being a powerful antioxidant, ALA may help stimulate insulin response, regulate blood glucose levels, and repair liver cells.

Tocotrienols

Vitamin E is comprised of two groups of molecules, notably tocopherols and tocotrienols. Each of these categories has four forms (alpha, beta, gamma, and delta-tocopherol, as well as alpha, beta, gamma and delta-tocotrienol). Scientific research is starting to focus on specific tocopherols and tocotrienols, rather than just "vitamin E." Nonetheless, the vitamin E most often referred to and sold in most stores is a synthetic form called d-alpha-tocopherol.

Isolated vitamin E, or d-alpha tocopherol, does not have good results in lowering the risk of heart attacks. However, a growing body of research suggests that the tocotrienols lower cholesterol and have potent chemopreventive effects, much like flavonoids. Tocotrienols are members of the vitamin E family. Like vitamin E, tocotrienols are potent antioxidants against lipid peroxidation (the damaging of fats by oxidation and free radical activity).[31] Human studies indicate that, in addition to their antioxidant activity, tocotrienols have other important functions, especially in maintaining a healthy cardiovascular system. Mohammad Minhajuddin, PhD of the University of Rochester and colleagues reported in the May 2005 issue of *Food and Chemical Toxicology* that tocotrienols from rice bran oil significantly lower total and low-density lipoprotein cholesterol (LDL).

Like vitamin E, tocotrienols may offer protection against hardening of the arteries (atherosclerosis) by preventing oxidative damage to LDL cholesterol (oxidation of LDL cholesterol is believed to be one of the triggering factors for atherosclerosis).

Tocotrienols are found primarily in the oil fraction of rice bran, palm fruit, barley, and wheat germ. Supplemental sources of tocotrienols are derived from rice bran oil and palm oil distillates. Tocotrienol supplements are available in capsules and tablets.

Fiber and Digestive Aids

Psyllium Supplement and other Natural Fiber

Unquestionably, soluble fiber, when taken as part of a regular diet, can lower your total and LDL cholesterol levels.[32] A good example is psyllium, which is a natural fiber (the same fiber used in Metamucil). Studies have repeatedly shown that psyllium lowers cholesterol when taken every day. You might stir it into orange juice, as this fruit has shown remarkable improvement in blood pressure.

Other excellent natural foods that lower cholesterol include whole oats (or oatmeal), beans, peas, rice bran, barley and certain fruits, such as oranges, strawberries, pears and apples. Certain vegetables like brussel sprouts and carrots are good sources of fiber.

PGX™

A company called Natural Factors Nutritional Products, Ltd. (known under the trade name "Natural Factors" and located in Canada) has a product called PGX™, which is a highly viscous fiber blend of glucomannan, xanthan, and alginate that may help lower LDL and total cholesterol. Even more important may be its ability to limit sugar absorption and the subsequent after-meal insulin spike. High after-meal blood glucose and insulin levels increase the risk of heart attacks significantly. When study subjects took just one gram of glucomannan before each meal, total cholesterol was reduced by 21.7 mg/dL and LDL was lowered by 14 mg/dL. The only side effect of this supplement is excessive gas, due to unabsorbed starches.

Essential Fatty Acids

Omega-3 Fatty Acids Contained in Fish Oil

As explained in Chapter 5, supplanting your diet with omega-3 fish oil capsules has shown the potential to reduce both the progression of cardiovascular disease and related mortality, including sudden cardiac death.

The fish-oil-based omega-3 fatty acids, which are really a form of polyunsaturated fat, consist of EPA and DHA. Plant foods and vegetable oils typically lack EPA and DHA, although some do contain varying amounts of alpha linolenic acid (ALA). Many vegetable oils are greatly enriched in the not so good omega-6 fatty acids (mainly as linoleic acid in corn, safflower, sunflower and soybean oils). However, as noted in earlier chapters, non-hydrogenated canola oil, ground flaxseed and walnuts are rich sources of ALA.

Many studies that I have reviewed seem to consistently conclude that despite all things being equal, or approximately equal in terms of cholesterol levels, people with a high ratio of omega-3 oil, have less risk of cardiovascular disease.[33] Stated another way, the degree to which you consume EPA and DHA (omega-3 fatty acids) is inversely related to levels of your LDL cholesterol, levels of the not so good omega-6 fatty acids, and your overall risk of coronary heart disease. After all the technical analysis is over and the "verdict is in" so to speak, consuming fish (up to 2-3 servings per week), or more ideally fish oil, appears to be associated with lower heart attack rates and death from cardiovascular disease.

Herbs

Garlic

This plant is mentioned in several places throughout this book. We first touched on its properties in a negative sense, when there was a suggestion that it could be one of the foods to which you could be sensitive in connection with triggering AFIB. If you are one of these people, I can definitely empathize with you as you are hereby given my special condolences. As you know, garlic not only gives food its wonderful flavor, but it is also a powerful antioxidant (containing vitamin A, vitamin C and selenium) and also has been used for a variety of ailments, such as the reduction of plaque buildup in your arteries, lowered levels of cholesterol and triglycerides, improved circulation, improved flexibility of the aorta (which pumps blood from the heart to the rest of your body), and as you will learn in the next chapter, a reduction in blood pressure.

The problem with garlic, however, is that in most cases it is overcooked and the beneficial ingredient, allicin, is destroyed. So, the best thing to do is to continue to cook flavorful foods and take garlic supplements in pill form undiminished by the cooking process.

Arjuna

Arjuna or *Terminalia arjuna* is an Indian medicinal plant. This unique herb helps maintain a healthy heart and supports immunity to bacterial infections, as well as reduces the effects of stress and nervousness.[34] Arjuna's ability to suppress your blood's absorption of lipids indicates that it has cholesterol-regulating properties. It reduces the level of triglycerides and cholesterol and has been reported to enhance the synthesis of LDL-apoprotein (apoB). Further, it inhibits the oxidation of LDL and accelerates the turnover of LDL in your liver. This enhances the elimination of oxidized cholesterol from your body.

The bark of arjuna is also useful to regulate blood pressure by increasing your blood supply to your bodily organs and tissues, and is particularly useful where there is a constriction or obstruction of the blood vessels. This means that arjuna has "anti-ischemic" properties and is quite effective in dealing with hypertension, especially where your cardiac rhythm is irregular or you have angina pains.

Lifestyle Changes

Exercise Regularly

Exercise decreases your bad LDL cholesterol and increases your "good" HDL cholesterol. If you are well-trained, your "good" HDL is increased considerably. Most population studies have shown that physical exercise is associated with a lower risk of coronary heart disease, and a sedentary life with a higher risk. It also seems plausible that a well-trained heart is better guarded against obstruction of the coronary vessels than a heart always working at low speed. A sedentary life may predispose you to a heart attack and, at the same time, lower the HDL/LDL ratio.

You must remember, however, if you exercise too hard, it can cause a heart attack if you had been sedentary and have a history of heart disease. In early 2005, the March/April issue of Psychosomatic Medicine published an interesting report where it was stated that exercise reduced the risk of heart attacks for healthy people but had the opposite effect on inactive cardiac patients who might be prejudicing their health by engaging in strenuous activities. The study revealed that people who seldom exercised were nearly seven times more likely to suffer a heart attack after engaging in strenuous activities over those who exercised more than three times a week.

The problem that we have with this conclusion is that if you suffered a heart attack after enduring some form of workout or physical exercise you might become fearful of engaging in exercise in the future. However, exercise prevents, and to a certain extent solves, a myriad of health problems like high blood pressure, stress, depression, breast and colon cancers, and osteoporosis, in addition to lowering cholesterol. If you are overweight, have high blood pressure, high cholesterol or diabetes, then you will want to consider a slowly building daily exercise program, working more and more each day and you will eventually see improvement. Use exercise like an elixir, a very natural, normal and needed bodily function, much like eating, sleeping and talking.

Strategy #6 in Chapter 5 discusses walking and how that is used to curtail arrhythmias. Well, the same strategy can be used for other ailments. Simply start walking slowly and easily and work your way up. It is very low impact and less irritating to your joints.

There is, however, one important point to note on the concept of exercise, training and heart health. In the late spring of 2005, a famous track and field star died of sudden cardiac arrest without warning. This condition affects many people who would least likely be impacted by this fatal disease. Studies have shown, particularly as reported on *Good Morning America* on May 12, 2005, that athletes (or anyone for that matter) who has a resting heart rate of greater than 75 beats per minute and/or whose heart rate after exercise comes down very slowly has a much greater risk of sudden cardiac arrest. It was interesting to note that one of the suggestions by a mainstream medical doctor to reduce the risks of heart problems like this was consume omega-3 fatty acids from fish oil!

Special Foods and Extracts

Raw almonds

A handful (1/4-1/2 cup) of raw almonds daily not only lowers cholesterol, but also lowers the dreaded genetic risk factor for coronary disease, *lipoprotein(a)*. Almonds also suppress abnormal spikes in blood sugar after eating and help prevent diabetes. They are tremendously filling and are great for sugar addicts who need to snack, since almonds take the edge off your sweet tooth.[35]

Policosanol

Policosanol is actually a beneficial natural supplement derived, surprisingly enough, from sugar cane. If you have healthy arteries, they are lined with a smooth layer of cells (those endothelial cells) so that your blood can race through with no resistance. One of the features of diseased arteries is that this layer becomes thick and overgrown with cells. As the artery narrows, blood flow slows down or is blocked completely. Policosanol was tested for its ability to stop the proliferation of these cells and the results came out favorably. Policosanol can also help maintain this smooth layer of cells.[36]

Policosanol is another natural supplement that can normalize your cholesterol as well or better than drugs, and without side effects. Efficacy and safety have been proven in numerous clinical trials, and it has been used by millions of people in other countries. Policosanol lowers your LDL cholesterol and raises your protective HDL cholesterol.

What makes policosanol exciting is that it has other actions against heart disease in addition to lowering cholesterol. For example, policosanol helps stop the formation of artery lesions.

One of policosanol's important actions is to inhibit the oxidation of LDL.[37] Oxidized LDL is dangerous as it promotes the destruction of blood vessels by creating inflammation. Oxidized LDL can also promote blood vessel destruction in your body, partly by interfering with HDL's protective effect.

Policosanol also inhibits the formation of clots, and may work well with aspirin in this respect. In a comparison of aspirin and policosanol, aspirin was better at reducing one type of platelet aggregation (clumping together of blood cells).[38] But, policosanol was better at inhibiting another type. A related effect is that significant reductions in the level of thromboxane occur in humans after two weeks of policosanol. Thromboxane is a blood vessel-constricting agent that contributes to abnormal platelet aggregation that can cause a heart attack or stroke.

And, there is another side benefit of policosanol. Unlike cholesterol-lowering drugs that can induce impotency, policosanol may have a libido-enhancing effect! Studies in male rats show that policosanol increases sexual activity without increasing testosterone. The same results appear to be true for monkeys, but the studies are too few to be definitive. Unfortunately, very high amounts of policosanol had to be taken to get these effects. But, the good news is that when you take policosanol at recommended doses, it doesn't interfere with your sex life, which gives it an advantage over many cholesterol-lowering drugs.

The Benefits of Wine Without the Downsides

No other beverage has attracted the attention of modern medicine like wine, particularly in connection with heart health. One glass of red wine per day is universally thought of as good for your heart because of its high antioxidant content, which acts to guard stores of nitric oxide (nitric oxide is a very good ally in terms of heart health and is discussed below and in the next section in greater detail).

However, drinking excessively tends to cause your blood vessels to become narrower and a myriad of other heart and liver related problems. Although it is most widely known for its benefits for your heart, wine has benefits against cancer, dementia, and other age-related diseases. Researchers in Denmark recently looked at 25,000 people to find out what drinking alcohol does to mortality and discovered that wine drinkers slash their overall risk of dying from any cause by about 40%.

What is excessive red wine consumption? Well, most experts would agree that more than two glasses per day is excessive. And even two glasses per day is not totally safe from the negative effects of excessive consumption occurring.

Chemists took wine apart years ago to find out what makes it tick. Basically, wine contains a host of plant compounds. Unfortunately, nobody paid much attention to *resveratrol* and some of the other beneficial components until a scientist tried to figure out why the French can eat so much fat and not get heart disease. It turns out that part of the answer to this "French paradox" is resveratrol found in red wine.

Why can a person eat a lot of fat, yet not get heart disease? One of the reasons is that the wine they drink contains resveratrol, which is a powerful antioxidant. Remember, low density lipoprotein (LDL) is a problem in heart disease. This is why vitamin E helps prevent heart problems – this vitamin scavenges (or cleans up) the radicals that *oxidize* this fat/protein. However, the kind of radicals that vitamin E blocks are not the only kind of free radicals people have to worry about. There are other types. In a study published in *Free Radical Research,* resveratrol was put to the test against vitamin E and a synthetic antioxidant.[39] All three were very good at scavenging artery-damaging radicals, but resveratrol emerged as the best defense against certain types of radicals. This points out the importance of using a multi-approach to antioxidants.

One of the serious complications of free radical damage is hardening and thickening of arteries.[40] Resveratrol is just one of the suggested treatments for this progressive process. Resveratrol's antioxidant action helps stop free radical damage and opens the arteries by enhancing nitric oxide, a bodily chemical.

Nitric oxide is a critical component of heart/artery function. It allows blood vessels to "relax," which enhances blood flow.[41] Studies have shown that in a high-cholesterol diet, nitric oxide is reduced by about a third. Resveratrol supplements significantly reversed the trend. In this respect, resveratrol is similar to Viagra, which also affects nitric oxide. However, whereas Viagra only affects small vessels, resveratrol affects the main arteries. So, as an added benefit of this cholesterol lowering suggestion, your sex life may be improved!

Finally, resveratrol also stops the proliferation of cells in blood vessels that narrow the arteries, and it also keeps blood cells from sticking together.[42] Both are very important for preventing heart attacks.

In short, resveratrol would necessarily have a tremendous counteractive impact on the negative aspects of LDL in your bloodstream. And, the good news is that you don't have to drink red wine if you don't want to, as resveratrol comes in a pill form. So, you can have all the benefits of red wine without having to worry about the alcohol, the sugar and the calories.

THE NATURAL CHOLESTEROL SOLUTION II – WHAT YOU SHOULD NOT DO

First, you should eliminate, or demonstrably reduce, your reliance on sugars and grain-based food products, like breads, cakes, muffins, cookies, etc. But, if you have to eat some grain based products, stay away from processed white flour items and focus more on whole grains, whole wheat flour. However, doing all this will inevitably create "side effects", in that your weight will start to normalize, elevated insulin levels will subside, your energy (and even your sexual energy) will increase, and your blood pressure and your triglycerides may go down. It is to be specifically noted that elevated insulin levels are one of the primary catalysts for raising cholesterol. (for a further, more in-depth analysis, see the chapter below on "Taking the Pressure Off, the Natural Blood Pressure Solution II – What You Should Not Do")

Second, avoid sunflower, corn, soy, safflower, canola, and other vegetable oils or products that contain these oils. Do not use hydrogenated or partially hydrogenated fats, margarine, vegetable oil, or shortening. These oils are loaded with omega-6 fats and will only worsen your omega-6/omega-3 ratio. Acceptable oils are a high quality extra virgin olive oil, coconut oil, avocados, and organic butter, or optimally organic butter from grass-fed livestock.

Generally, if you have the typical American diet, you are consuming very worrisome levels of omega-6 fats. This means that you should greatly reduce the omega-6 fatty acids you are now consuming and increase your intake of omega-3 fatty acids.

Another way to improve your omega-6/omega-3 ratio is to change the type of meat you are eating. You could consume more game meat like venison, or other game animals that are raised exclusively on grass. However, these are hard to find and generally more expensive than beef. Since nearly all cattle are grain fed before slaughter, if you eat most traditionally raised beef, it will typically worsen you omega-6/omega-3 ratio.

To get the necessary omega-3 fatty acids, you should consider eating meat that is allowed to roam free on the range, commonly known as "free-range", and in the case of cattle, it is to be grass-fed. Sadly, it is rare to be able to buy this kind of beef at your local food store. Even though it might say grass fed beef does not mean it will be grass fed beef, mainly because they are fed grain for several months before slaughter, notwithstanding the cattle may have had grass the majority of their life. You can tell good grass fed beef from the way it feels in your hands – much less greasy and slippery. And, unfortunately, this is the "rub" with grass fed meat – it is generally less tender when comparing it with artificially and excessively fattened grain fed beef.

___

Chapter 8 taught you that cholesterol is something you actually want to have, as it assists in the efficient operation of many bodily functions. Cholesterol, in and of itself, does not cause heart disease, but is rather a powerful weapon against free radical damage in the blood and a repair material that actually heals the damage that occurs within your arteries.

In order to get to a certain place in your body to carry out one of its many functions, cholesterol uses lipoproteins to carry the cholesterol around. The high density lipoprotein (HDL) carries cholesterol from your tissues to your liver, and low density lipoproteins (LDL), which is the vast majority of your total cholesterol, away from your liver to your cells. Your body goes haywire when the LDLs carrying cholesterol is directed to your blood vessel walls that have been damaged by certain types of injurious chemical reactions, notably free radicals. These chemical reactions are exacerbated when you have excessive cholesterol. In other words, your risks are higher because your have excessive amounts – not that LDL is the sole cause. HDL is good because it helps keep the chemical reactions from occurring and also helps keep cholesterol from attaching itself to existing plaque.

Cholesterol, in and of itself, is not bad for you. However, when combined with bad eating habits and bad lifestyle, cholesterol turns into a bad thing. But, it is not the cholesterol that is the culprit. Rather, it is the underlying free radical activity that causes the problems with the chemical composition and bodily processing of cholesterol. In short, cholesterol has been framed by the big business marketers because it has been convenient and profitable to do so.

In reality, high levels of cholesterol does not cause of heart disease, but is more of a marker of its potential to cause heart disease in your body, under certain conditions. The drug industry has literally pounced on the opportunity to create one of the biggest distortions in American medical history by convincing almost everyone that cholesterol is bad and it must be lowered easily and quickly through the use of prescription drugs. What is conveniently ignored is the very significant negative side effects of these drugs.

Managing your cholesterol in an objective, knowledgeable manner through natural means will allow you to maintain your health and prevent premature death from cardiovascular disease. You can maintain desirable cholesterol levels through such natural strategies (as an alternative to statin prescription drugs) by combining lifestyle modifications, exercise, natural supplements and dietary strategies. The lack of negative side effects (that are otherwise associated with the statin drugs) makes such natural strategies especially attractive for maintaining healthy cholesterol levels.

Chapter 9
Reduce the Risk of Stroke:
Looking Beyond Cholesterol

"Thousands and thousands of people have studied disease. Almost no one has studied health."

—Adelle Davis

I have previously discussed the conventional risks for plaque or deposits in your arteries and veins – high LDL (bad) cholesterol, low HDL (good) cholesterol resulting from free radical activity and/or bad genes, smoking, obesity and improper fat intake. Another factor is diabetes, but that is the subject of an entire book. When it comes to heart health, fats and cholesterol are not the top enemies as I have preached herein *ad nauseum*. In fact, your body needs them to stay healthy. What fats and cholesterol actually do is <u>measure</u> the physiological process that <u>precedes</u> the plaque build-up. And, it is because of this atherosclerotic plaque that we have the third leading cause of death in this country – stroke.

Stroke is a humbling illness, reducing an active vibrant human being to a helpless, immobile creature. It can destroy or impair crucial functions such as speech, swallowing, walking, and bowel and bladder control. One person dies every three minutes due to stroke. If you have a stroke, there is a 25% chance that you will die within a year. And, all this does not happen cheaply. In 2004 alone, the direct and indirect costs of stroke in the U.S. were $53.6 billion according to reports from the American Heart Association.

Stroke does not happen overnight. In fact, it takes many decades to develop. Luckily, today's technology can detect stroke years before the disease can take effect. As with most of the illnesses discussed in this book (not to mention most other illnesses as well), the mainstream medical practitioner focuses on the stroke <u>after</u> it happens rather than on preventing it in the first place. They focus on sur-

150

gery or stints rather than preventative solutions and care, which I believe to be a glaring failure of our healthcare system.

So, how does stroke develop? What can be done to screen and diagnose the risk of a stroke for you? And, what nutritional techniques and lifestyle changes can you make to essentially de-plaque yourself? Chapter 9 leads the way to these answers.

HOW YOU CAN DEVELOP STROKE

Stroke occurs when some portion of your brain is deprived of oxygen because your blood is not getting it there. How does this happen? Well, this occurs because there is a blockage caused by some debris lodged within an artery. This blockage is essentially the same sort of plaque that accumulates in your arteries and causes heart attacks.

The blockages that typically occur to produce stroke are in the carotid arteries located on both sides of your neck. There are other areas (like the aorta, which is the main artery that leads blood out from your heart), but these are the main ones.

So, the question now becomes, how does plaque develop and how does it get in a position to cause stroke? Well, you just learned that plaque forms within arteries and blood vessels when an injury to the lining of one of your blood vessels or arteries occurs. When this happens, your white blood cells, LDL cholesterol and other bodily fluids flood the site of the injury and inflammation occurs. The artery or blood vessel lining reacts by adding layers of elastin and collagen fibers, further restricting the flow of blood. This is how plaque is formed. If you have a poor diet, don't exercise, have high cholesterol and/or are overweight, this plaque can grow and become unstable, break off and travel to your brain. But, this is not the only problem that can occur from fragmented plaque. The little bits and pieces that break off can interfere with your flowing blood and cause blood clot formation, which can also travel to your brain and cause stroke.

HOW TO DETERMINE IF YOU ARE AT RISK FOR STROKE

Tests to Determine if There is Plaque Build-up

First, new imaging technologies are becoming more accurate and accessible all the time. Computed tomography scanning (CT scans) and magnetic resonance imaging (MRI) are developing areas to detect stroke on a non-invasive basis. The problem is that they are typically (but not always) used on people who have already suffered a stroke.

There is one test that is used in connection with preventative maintenance and that is a process known as carotid ultrasound. This test is harmless, painless and non-invasive and relatively simple to perform. The process detects and measures plaque fragmentation potential as well as your potential for developing plaque even if you don't have it yet. The only problem with this test is the results. Many interpreters will only report whether plaque is present or not. However, more significant is a measurement called *"carotid intimamedia thickness"*, which determines your body wide predisposition for developing atherosclerotic plaque. If you have this test performed, try to obtain a reading in this connection as well. Most of the literature that I have read on this test suggests that a good measure is to have an *intima-media thickness* of less than 1.0 mm. This carotid ultrasound test is not expensive and is clearly worth the cost.

Tests to Determine Your Potential for Developing Stroke

There are several markers that can measure the likelihood of your developing stroke.

High C-reactive Protein and Homocysteine Levels

C-reactive protein (CRP) and homocysteine, are actually two very excellent markers for heart disease that are frequently overlooked.[43] They are good markers because they can spot the problem early on. Homocysteine is a measure of oxidation in your blood vessels, and C-reactive protein is an early measure of inflammation. Actually, they are better predictors of heart disease than cholesterol or any other factor!

Increased levels of CRP indicate damage and inflammation and a higher risk for stroke. Increased risk begins at levels above 0.5 mg/L. High CRP also predicts more rapidly growing plaque. High homocysteine appears to be a direct irritant to the lining of the blood vessel walls. By lowering your homocysteine and CRP levels, you can prevent further damage and even heal the damage that's already been done.

Hypertension

A simple blood pressure check can serve to measure the risk of having stroke as there is a good correlation between high blood pressure and stroke. Chapter 10 outlines in great detail the causes and natural cures for high blood pressure, so we will not replicate that discussion here. Suffice it to say, considerable research documents the power of lowering your blood pressure in helping to prevent stroke.

Diabetes and Metabolic Syndrome

Being overweight can readily lead to diabetes (which can cause plaque to accumulate and particularly cause carotid plaque to grow) as well as a condition known as metabolic syndrome, which consists of excessive abdominal fat, high blood pressure, low HDL, high triglycerides, and resistance to insulin. Sound like 70% of American males over the age of 40? Well, it seems like it is. But, in reality metabolic syndrome is largely an epidemic impacting one-third of all adults due to sedentary lifestyles and poor food choices.

Special Lipoprotein Measurements

At the outset of this chapter we noted that there were other, more significant markers of heart disease and stroke than high cholesterol. One such marker involves various abnormalities amongst your lipoproteins. When we talk about lipoproteins, what comes to mind are the HDLs and the LDLs already discussed. Well, that is not exactly what I am talking about here.

Recall that lipoproteins are essentially proteins that carry fat around in the blood and certain of them actually cause plaque to grow. But, this includes various sub-types of lipoproteins like (i) *small LDL particles* (which encourage carotid plaque to grow more than the large LDL particles we have been talking about so far), (ii) *intermediate density lipoproteins* (IDL) (which measure how effectively fat is cleared out after a large meal (if you have high levels of IDL it can create plaque high in soft unstable fat that makes it more prone to rupture), (iii) *LDL particle number, also known as apolipoprotein B* (which I discussed earlier, is known to be a the actual count of LDL particles in the blood and is superior to LDL and total cholesterol as a predictor of heart disease and stroke), and (iv) *lipoprotein (a)* (a factor that promotes blood clotting and constricted arteries, increases the dangers of cholesterol and promotes accelerated plaque growth).

Fibrinogen

Our old foe, fibrinogen, once again comes into the discussion about stroke. This blood clotting protein does something more than promoting carotid plaque – it actually assists in the formation of unstable plaques. These plaques are more inflamed and are thinner, which makes them more prone to rupture. Pay attention to this valuable marker when you get your medical check-ups.

NATURAL, SAFE WAYS TO COMBAT STROKE

How do you reduce the risk of stroke – without resorting to drugs or invasive medical procedures?

First, undertake a regimen of the supplements mentioned in Chapter 5, notably fish oil (to reduce inflammation, reduce plaque and the instability thereof, lower triglycerides, and provide modest anti-coagulation effects). New studies about omega-3 fatty acids are so impressive that even the Federal government has stated that fish oil can help save lives. In a report issued on April 22, 2004, an agency of the National Institutes of Health stated: "fish oil can help reduce deaths from heart disease."

Secondly, consume 100-200 mg of CoQ10 per day (to reduce blood pressure and strengthen your heart), and magnesium (to also lower blood pressure).

Thirdly, take a good multivitamin with potent levels of vitamin C, vitamin E and the B vitamins, particularly B2, B6 and B12, along with folic acid.

Fourth, take a supplement called *trimethylglycine* (TMG for short), which I will explain in greater detail below.

Fifth, use garlic freely (provided you do not have an arrhythmia sensitivity to it) as it protects your blood from attack, reduces arterial plaque, acts as an anti-thrombotic agent (prevents blood clotting), lowers blood pressure and decreases the accumulation of cholesterol in the vascular walls. And, if that is not enough garlic has shown to be an excellent antioxidant and free radical scavenger.

Sixth, there are a number of supplements to correct metabolic syndrome. If you are overweight, change your eating habits and exercise at least 45 minutes four days a week. Some weight loss ideas are contained in Chapter 10 on controlling blood pressure, like white bean extract and glucomannan, which are two of the ingredients in PGX™ discussed throughout this book. This supplement blocks intestinal absorption of carbohydrates by at least two-thirds and, when taken before meals, absorbs many times its weight in water and thereby fills the stomach, causing you to eat less. Also, consider supplementation with an adrenal hormone called DHEA, which is essential to maintaining physical stamina, mood, muscle mass in men, and libido in women. Studies have shown results in reduced abdominal fat particularly from insulin resistance, a risk factor for stroke. One other supplement is pectin (which most people are familiar with in the form of apple pectin). Pectin provides a good feeling of fullness while at the same time lowers cholesterol and slows the release of sugars. Outside of apples, pectin is abundant in citrus rinds and green vegetables.

How do these nutrients all work together to prevent stroke? Since you have read Part I of this book, you should have a fairly good understanding of the benefits of fish oil, CoQ10 and magnesium. And, if you are not a biochemist, just rely on the fact that they do an excellent job of reducing the risk of stroke and heart disease and skip the next three paragraphs.

However, if you are technically minded, consider that elevated homocysteine can be reduced (or detoxified) in two ways. The most common pathway is to enhance a chemical process in your body called "methylation." Enhancing methylation improves health and slows premature and, perhaps, normal aging. Methylation lowers dangerous homocysteine levels, thus lowering the risk of heart disease and stroke.

A potent remethylation agent is the TMG that was noted above, which stands for trimethylglycine. TMG is the most effective methylation enhancing agent known.

TMG is extracted from sugar beets. It has a distinctive taste that is mildly sweet with a mild aftertaste. TMG is also known as glycine betaine. Some vitamin companies confuse "betaine hydrochloride" with glycine betaine (TMG). Betaine HCL does not provide the methylation enhancement of TMG and could elevate stomach acidity in some people. There are no reports of side effects with TMG other than brief muscle tension headaches if it is taken in large quantities without food.

Choline is another "methyl donor" that helps to lower elevated homocysteine levels. However, choline only enhances remethylation in the liver and kidney, which is why it is so important to take adequate amounts of remethylating factors such as folic acid and vitamin B12 to protect the brain and the heart. The published literature emphasizes that folic acid and vitamin B12 are critical nutrients in the remethylation (detoxification) pathway of homocysteine.

For many people, the daily intake of 500 mg of TMG, 800 mcg of folic acid, 1000 mcg of vitamin B12, 250 mg of choline, 250 mg of inositol, 30 mg of zinc, and 100 mg of vitamin B6 will keep homocysteine levels in a safe range. But the only way to really know is to have your blood tested to make sure your homocysteine levels are under 7. If homocysteine levels are too high, then up to 6 grams of TMG may be needed along with higher amounts of other remethylation cofactors. Some people with cystathione-B synthase deficiencies will require 500 mg a day or more of vitamin B6 to reduce homocysteine to a safe level. For the prevention of cardiovascular disease, you would want your homocysteine blood level to be under 7. For the prevention of aging, some people have suggested that an even lower level is desirable, but more research needs to be done before any scientific conclusions can be reached.

However, there really is no safe "normal range" for homocysteine. According to Circulation, the American Heart Association's journal (November 15, 1995), while commercial laboratories state that normal homocysteine can range from 5 to 15 micromoles per liter of blood, epidemiological data reveal that homocysteine levels above 6.3 cause a steep, progressive risk of heart attack. So, when you get tested, be cautious and critical of the results.

In chapter 9 you learned that there are more and more ways to guard against and reliably measure arterial plaque build-up. And, there are some very reliable tests to determine if you are at greater risk for stroke and if there is plaque build-up already.

In order to effectively prevent stroke, you should engage in a relatively multifaceted approach incorporating an all out attack on metabolic syndrome, C-reactive protein, homocysteine levels and certain subcategories of lipoproteins. As we have continually stressed, fish oil is your best place to start and is the most beneficial nutrient you can take to guard against stroke. Other nutrients target a certain specific risk factor for stroke, which can be individualized based upon your particular circumstances.

Chapter 10
Take the Pressure Off Your Blood

"Your body is the baggage you must carry through life. The more excess baggage the shorter the trip."

—E. Glasgow

Chapter 10 discusses one of the most common ailments for people all over the world, particularly Americans – high blood pressure. You will learn about the gravity and tremendous expanse of the problem. You will discover what blood pressure is all about and what happens when you have high blood pressure. You will also be fascinated to learn how blood pressure can build up as well as the factors causing blood pressure to build up. And, a discussion of high blood pressure would not be complete without going into detail on prescription drugs as compared with natural strategies to curb elevated blood pressure levels.

THE GRIM STATISTICS

High blood pressure is an even stronger predictor of cardiovascular risk than high cholesterol. Scientific studies directly correlate high blood pressure with decreased longevity. Yet, most mainstream physicians and most Americans generally ignore this risk until life-threatening hypertension has already developed.

If you do not have high blood pressure, you will feel fine and typically take for granted the flow of your blood through your heart and your arteries. However, if you have high blood pressure, you probably ask yourself, "why me", "why am I so unlucky." If it's any consolation you are far from alone. Anyone can develop high blood pressure, but some are more likely to get it than others. Heredity plays a role. If your parents or grandparents had high blood pressure, your risk may be increased.

Fifty million Americans aged 6 and older have high blood pressure. Americans now 55 or over face a 90% chance of developing high blood pressure, or hypertension, a major risk factor for heart attacks, strokes, congestive heart failure, circulatory failure, kidney disease, and loss of vision. If you are not one of them, you likely will be eventually. Unfortunately, most mainstream physicians and their patients ignore this risk until life-threatening hypertension has already developed. To be sure, consider the following statistics.

One in five Americans (and one in four adults) has high blood pressure. In general, more men than women have high blood pressure. And, the number of both men and women with high blood pressure increases rapidly in older age groups. More than half of all Americans over the age of 65 (including 75% of women and 64% of men over age 75) have high blood pressure.

So, again, you are far from alone if you have high blood pressure. The important thing is to be proactive in knowing what blood pressure is all about, why your pressure is high and what you can do about it – without prescription drugs, without invasive procedures and without surgery.

WHAT IS BLOOD PRESSURE

So, you have obviously heard about high blood pressure. But, what is blood pressure all about in the first place?

Blood is carried from your heart to all parts of your body in vessels, which by now you probably know are called arteries. Blood pressure is the force of the blood pushing against the walls of the arteries. Each time your heart beats (about 60-70 times a minute at rest), it pumps out blood into your arteries. Your blood pressure is at its highest when the heart beats, pumping the blood. This is called systolic pressure. When your heart is at rest, between beats, your blood pressure falls. This is the diastolic pressure.

Blood pressure is always given as these two numbers, the systolic and diastolic pressures. Both are important. Usually they are written one above or before the other, such as 120/80 mmHg. The top number is the systolic and the bottom the diastolic. When the two measurements are written down, the systolic pressure is the first or top number, and the diastolic pressure is the second or bottom number (for example, 120/80). If your blood pressure is 120/80, you say that it is "120 over 80."

Blood pressure changes during the day. It is lowest as you sleep and rises when you get up. It also can rise when you are excited, nervous, or active.

Still, for most of your waking hours, your blood pressure stays pretty much the same when you are sitting or standing still. According to the National High Blood Pressure Education Program Coordinating Committee – a coalition of 39 major professional, public and voluntary organizations and seven federal agencies, your blood pressure measurement should be lower than 120/80. When the level stays high, 140/90 or higher, you have high blood pressure. Both numbers are important. If one or both numbers are usually high, you have high blood pressure. With high blood pressure, the heart works harder, your arteries take a beating, and your chances of a stroke, heart attack, and kidney problems are greater.

WHAT HAPPENS WHEN YOU HAVE HIGH BLOOD PRESSURE

Simply put, when your blood pressure is high, your heart has to work harder than normal, which puts both the heart and the arteries under a greater strain.

When your heart has to work harder for an extended time, it tends to enlarge. When your blood pressure is too high, your heart has to work progressively harder to pump enough blood and oxygen to your body's organs and tissues to meet their needs. The heart muscle stretches and thickens, and the heart stops functioning properly. A significantly enlarged heart has a hard time meeting the demands put on it and can fail.

When your blood pressure is too high, your arteries become scarred, hardened and less elastic. This occurs to some degree in all of us as we age, but elevated blood pressure speeds this process, which is called "hardening of the arteries" or atherosclerosis.

If your arteries become hardened or narrowed, they may be unable to supply the amount of blood the body's organs need. If your organs do not get enough oxygen and nutrients, they cannot function properly. There is also a risk that a blood clot may lodge in one of your arteries narrowed by atherosclerosis, depriving part of your body of its normal blood supply.

If your arteries that supply blood to the heart become clogged, blood flow to parts of your heart is slowed. When one vessel is completely closed off, blood ceases to flow to part of your heart, and portions of the heart muscle are damaged. This is what is known as a classic heart attack.

As noted earlier in the previous chapter, if the blood vessels in your brain progressively narrow, a stroke may occur. This happens when blood flow becomes inadequate, your brain cells are robbed of oxygen, and they die. Narrowing of your vessels also leads to a situation where a blood clot cannot move through your arteries, thereby blocking the flow of blood and deprives the tissue of oxygen located beyond the clot. About 80% of strokes are caused by the blockage of an artery in the neck or brain. People who suffer a stroke often are left with paralysis on one side of the body and loss of speech.

The primary function of your kidneys is to filter toxic chemicals from your blood. This process is accomplished in specialized structures inside your kidneys. The blood pressure of the vessels inside these filtering structures is critical for their proper functioning. When your arteries are narrowed and thickened by high blood pressure, blood flow to your kidney's filtering structures is reduced, and they cease to function properly. The amount of fluid that your kidneys can filter is reduced, leading to kidney failure. As a result, toxic materials build up in the body and you would need to undergo dialysis, which is the use of a machine as an artificial kidney. In fact, you may ultimately need a kidney transplant.

Your kidneys have their own feedback mechanism to maintain optimum blood pressure to assure its proper functioning. For example, when this internal mechanism senses that your blood pressure is too low, it tries to compensate by actually raising blood pressure, which begins a deadly spiral of higher and higher pressure.

The damage to blood vessels caused by high blood pressure leads to hundreds of thousands of heart attacks and strokes each year. Moreover, people with high blood pressure have a much greater risk of developing adult-onset diabetes, and most people with diabetes sustain their greatest harm from the hypertension that frequently accompanies it. Not surprisingly, high blood pressure is an even stronger predictor of cardiovascular risk than high cholesterol.

HOW BLOOD PRESSURE CAN BUILD UP AND GO DOWN

To a degree, understanding how blood pressure is regulated is important for you to gain a greater degree of control in its impact on your life. Think of blood pressure like your shower in the morning. The water pressure can be increased in two ways – either by opening the holes in your showerhead and letting more water out, or by tightening the holes of the showerhead and increasing the resistance to the outflow of water. In exactly the same manner, the blood pressure is dependent on two things: the amount of blood being pumped by the heart (this is called the "*cardiac output*") and the resistance to flow (this is called the "*peripheral resistance*"). The latter is regulated largely by the diameter of the small arteries (once again, they are called "*arterioles*"), which have muscle fibers in their walls, and like the showerhead in your bathroom that you can constrict and dilate. This means that when your blood pressure goes up it can do so in three ways, either by an increase in the cardiac output or by constriction of the arterioles, or by a combination of the two. When you exercise, your pressure goes up because of an increased cardiac output, because the muscles need a greater flow of blood. If you put your hand in iced water your pressure also goes up, but in this case it's purely from constriction of the arterioles.

Your brain plays a major role in the regulation of your blood flow as well. This occurs through two sets of nerves, which act in opposite ways. I have alluded to these systems above, but a brief review would be helpful. Recall the sympathetic nervous system, which causes the heart to speed up, while the other, the parasympathetic system, makes it slow down. For example, when you exercise, your heart rate starts to go up at the beginning of exercise. This results from a combination of decreased parasympathetic and increased sympathetic nerve activity. The parasympathetic nerves are mainly involved in the regulation of the heart, while the sympathetic nervous system also controls the flow that occurs within your blood vessels, and regulates the "fight or flight response" characterized by an increased cardiac output and blood pressure. Historically, your body was essentially designed, in part, for the appropriate preparation in connection with vigorous physical exercise, whether it be fighting or fleeing from a foe. However, in modern times our threats are more often psychological rather than physical, and this pattern of response may be less appropriate for dealing with them. As an example, in times of mental stress, your heart pounds, your skin becomes sweaty and you have demonstrable anxiety, yet you have not undergone any physical exertion.

What is happening is that your sympathetic nerves (those associated with the fight/stress response) are transmitting their message to the muscle cells of your heart and arteries by releasing a chemical called "*norepinephrine*" (this is sometimes also called "*noradrenaline*") from the nerve terminals. These terminals rest on the surface of the muscle cells of your heart and arterioles and basically tell your muscles to work harder. Now, if you are wondering, "is this where you get the term 'adrenaline' or 'adrenaline rush', you are correct.

Technically, the norepinephrine goes to specific places on your muscle cells, which in turn sends a chemical signal to the inside of your cell to initiate the process of contraction. These places inside your cells are called "*adrenergic receptors*" and are of two sorts – alpha and beta. The alpha-receptors are mainly situated on the muscle cells in the walls of your arterioles (the arteries that branch out from your main arteries), and when stimulated cause your muscle to contract, and hence your arteriole to constrict. Beta receptors are located in several different sites, the most important ones being in your heart, where they stimulate both the strength and speed of contraction, and in your kidney, where they stimulate the release of a very important chemical that your body produces, called *"renin"*, which is also important in the regulation of blood pressure, as more particularly described below. So, to review – alpha receptors deals with your arterioles and beta receptors deal with your heart and kidney.

If you are given blood pressure medicine, these adrenergic receptors are what the medicine is aimed at. The medicines have some structural similarity to, and are designed to work on, the same general principle as, norepinephrine, which enables them to bind to these adrenergic receptors. But, unlike norepinephrine, they do not stimulate the receptor to trigger muscle contraction, and they also prevent the norepinephrine from stimulating the receptors. Hence, the drugs are appropriately called "blocking agents" because they block the effect the norepinephrine has on your adrenergic receptors. So, when you hear of the terms "alpha blockers" and "beta blockers", which is what they mean. The net effect of both alpha and beta blockers is to lower blood pressure, alpha blockers by dilating your arterioles, and beta blockers by lowering cardiac output and shutting off renin release in your kidneys. These drugs are given to people who have had a heart attack to prevent future problems and people who are about to undergo surgery to prevent complications during surgery like AFIB.

The muscle cells in your arterioles are structurally and functionally different from your heart muscle and the muscles in the rest of your body, and are referred to as "smooth muscle cells." In addition to the norepinephrine process discussed above, the contraction of your arterioles depends on the amount of calcium inside the cell. In fact, the contraction process is triggered by a small amount of calcium passing into your cells through minute pores called *"calcium channels."* The entrance to these channels can be blocked by another group of agents (which have been developed into prescription drugs), which are called "calcium channel blockers." These drugs work by slowing the rate at which calcium passes into the heart muscle and into the vessel walls. By relaxing the smooth muscles around the arteries and widening the vessels, more of your blood can flow more smoothly. This can lower your blood pressure, slow down your heart rate and can even relieve angina.

Another major mechanism for controlling blood pressure is *"angiotensin-converting enzyme inhibitors"* (also known as "ACE inhibitors", which is part of your *renin-angiotensin* system). I touched on renin previously. Well, renin is a chemical that is secreted by your kidneys, and circulates in your blood. Renin has no effect on your blood pressure itself, but it leads to the formation of another chemical – *angiotensin I*. As renin circulates through your lungs, angiotensin I is converted into *angiotensin II* by the *angiotensin converting enzyme (ACE)*. Angiotensin II exerts a very powerful constrictor effect on your arterioles, and thus can raise your blood pressure. Angiotensin II has a second effect, however, which makes it even more potent. It acts on your adrenal gland to release a hormone called *aldosterone*, which in turn acts on your kidney and causes it to retain sodium. This also tends to raise your blood pressure. One of the normal functions of the renin-angiotensin system is as a defense mechanism to maintain your blood pressure in situations such as hemorrhage or extreme salt depletion. A low blood pressure and a low amount of salt passing through your kidney are two of the three factors which stimulate your kidney to release renin, the third being the sympathetic nervous system. So, the ACE inhibitors block the renin-angiotensin action and cause a reduction in your blood pressure. And, or course, if you have not guessed by now, ACE inhibitors are prescription drugs.

HYPERTENSION AND HOW IT AFFECTS BLOOD PRESSURE

Many people think the term hypertension means high blood pressure. However, that is actually not the case, as hypertension is merely a cause of high blood pressure, albeit the major cause. In fact, in more than 95% of people who have high blood pressure, the underlying cause is listed as "*essential hypertension.*" What this means is that there is no obvious cause for the hypertension, such as a blocked artery. (The other 5% of people, where there is an identifiable cause, have "*secondary hypertension*", consistent with the definition of secondary high blood pressure). Basically what essential hypertension means is that it's there, and we don't know exactly why. And, the hypertension simply refers to the tension of pressure in the arteries; it does not, as many people might think, refer to nervous tension (although there is some recent evidence that nervous tension may contribute to its development).

The causes of essential hypertension are not well understood. However, there are several mechanisms involved, and these factors play different roles in different individuals. Probably about 50% of hypertension is genetic – that is, you inherit some tendency to have high blood pressure from your parents, just as you do your height, and the other 50% is environmental. There are almost certainly many different genes involved, and scientists are busily searching to identify them.

ENVIRONMENTAL FACTORS ASSOCIATED WITH HIGH BLOOD PRESSURE

As noted, for the vast majority of high blood pressure cases, the cause is really not known. However, it is significant to look at a number of environmental and other factors so that we can better understand the condition and have a better insight into the potential causes for any one particular condition.

There is a lot of controversy as to what are the important environmental factors. Some studies have shown that people who live in traditional non-westernized societies who later move to a modern city adopting a western lifestyle show a marked increase of blood pressure, which may be caused by the change in diet (salt intake typically goes up), or by stress, or probably both. Similarly, when people move from a traditional rural life to the big cities, their blood pressure goes up, but whether this is from stress or a change of diet is uncertain.

Of the environmental factors that cause high blood pressure, the two leading ones are thus stress and diet. One reason why we can't be sure about their exact roles is that both are complex and hard to measure. From a practical standpoint, what is stressful to one person is not necessarily so stressful to another. And trying to score your level of stress so that we can compare it with another person's is obviously very arbitrary. Diet is in principal easier to measure, but people vary what they eat from day to day, and there are almost certainly many ingredients other than salt and calories, which affect the blood pressure, which we are only just beginning to understand.

High blood pressure is also associated with the lack of potassium and magnesium in the diet, especially in relation to salt intake. Other lifestyle factors that may play a role are smoking and coffee and alcohol consumption. There is also some evidence that contamination from heavy metals such as lead, mercury, and cadmium can promote high blood pressure.

PANIC ATTACKS, BLOOD PRESSURE AND IRREGULAR HEARTBEATS

While there is a connection between panic attacks and hypertension, it does not tell us which is the chicken and which is the egg. The fact that the hypertension started before a panic attack makes it unlikely that the attacks were the direct cause of the hypertension, however. Other studies have shown that blood pressure goes up during an attack, but it comes down again when the attack is over. What causes these attacks remains somewhat of a mystery.

If you have suffered through PVCs, PACs or AFIB, your symptoms are often worse because you are suffering from another medical phenomena – panic attacks. According to miscellaneous psychology glossaries, the definition of a panic attack is "a discrete period of intense fear or discomfort involving at least four of the following symptoms":

- Shortness of breath or smothering symptoms
- Dizziness, unsteadiness or faintness
- Palpitations or rapid heart beats
- Trembling or shaking
- Sweating
- Choking
- Nausea or stomach upset
- Depersonalization or feeling of unreality
- Numbness or tingling
- Hot flushes or chills
- Chest pin or discomfort
- Fear of dying
- Fear of going crazy or losing control

Usually, palpitations, shaking or shivering, fear of dying and fear of going crazy or losing control are known to accompany the more benign arrhythmias. Interestingly, studies have shown that panic attacks are more prevalent in people with high blood pressure. In most patients the panic attacks started after the hypertension.

In the case of a person with a history of arrhythmias, a panic attack is to be expected, although the condition has some interrelationship with a generally anxious personality. Nevertheless, if you have PCs or AFIB, you clearly know that a panic attack is often hard to fight. But, with the information contained in Part I, hopefully you will have a better understanding of the inter-workings of the various benign heart arrhythmias that affect millions of Americans just like you. Realize that your condition is typically not life threatening, it should pass, and there will be a brighter day.

ARE YOU A SLAVE TO YOUR BLOOD PRESSURE MEDICINE

Treating high blood pressure only with prescription medications can be expensive and may cause potentially dangerous side effects. With over 50 million Americans having high blood pressure and with the relatively recent changes to the guidelines on hypertension, that number is sure to rise. Pharmaceutical companies have introduced a large number of medications to combat this deadly health condition and in fact, studies have shown that a significant portion of total prescribed medications in the U.S. are blood pressure medicines. With drug costs rising at an annual rate of at least 12% a year since 1993, you, particularly if you are elderly, can end up spending thousands of dollars a year on prescription medications to control your blood pressure. While the majority of prescription drugs that are used to control hypertension work well, they can have troublesome to potentially deadly side effects according to the American Heart Association's website (www.americanheart.org), such as hyperglycemia (high blood glucose), tinnitus (constant ringing or buzzing in the ears), impotence, kidney damage and many others, including heart failure itself!

Mainstream healthcare providers and practitioners would have you believe (and probably believe it themselves) that expensive prescription medications are the only proven way to combat hypertension. However, the truth is that there are some supplements that can help keep your blood pressure below that all important 120/80 figure.

Before considering the active *treatment* of hypertension, the even greater need for *prevention* of disease should be recognized. Yet mainstream medical doctor are usually content to wait for high blood pressure to develop in their patient and then treat it. Few doctors actively advise patients about how to prevent the disorder from occurring in the first place.

For people with hypertension who are hesitant to use expensive prescription medications with potentially significant side effects, there are recognized non-drug strategies that may significantly help in controlling high blood pressure. Just by incorporating lifestyle modifications such as dietary changes, smoking cessation and weight loss, blood pressure can be brought down and controlled in a significant number of people.

Being proactive relative to keeping your blood pressure in check is seemingly vital to maintaining a healthy cardiovascular system, whether or not you are a person who experiences arrhythmias. There are certain natural supplements you can take and lifestyle changes you can make to enable you to prevent high blood pressure if you don't have the condition. And, if you do have it, you can achieve reduced blood pressure readings and a more relaxed new you.

Prevention is even more important today because a blood pressure of 120/80 mm Hg (systolic/diastolic) is not good enough anymore, since, as I stated earlier, that reading is on the uppermost end of what is considered to be normal. Thus, you must do what you can to keep your blood pressure low instead of waiting for it to creep up over the years. You must be proactive because many people have a genetic tendency toward hypertension. Even if you have such a tendency, this does not mean you are powerless. As with predispositions toward developing diabetes or elevated cholesterol, much can be done to prevent hypertension from occurring or to modify its severity if it does occur. So, let's consider the following proactive measures!

THE NATURAL BLOOD PRESSURE SOLUTION I – WHAT YOU SHOULD DO

Minerals

Increase Your Mineral Intake of Magnesium, Calcium and Potassium

Sufficient intake of the minerals calcium, potassium, and magnesium is important for you to control your blood pressure. There have been numerous studies showing that changing to a diet high in these vitally important minerals, or taking them as supplements, can significantly help control hypertension. Numerous studies over the past 15 years have focused on the association between calcium, potassium and magnesium intake and hypertension. The Joint National Committee on Prevention, Detection, Evaluation, and Treatment of High Blood Pressure recommends adequate amounts of potassium in the diet, along with other measures such as dietary calcium and weight loss, to prevent the development of high blood pressure. The National Heart, Lung, and Blood Institute (NHLBI) conducted a series of studies relative to reducing high blood pressure through dietary means. One study called "DASH", stands for dietary approaches to stop hypertension. The DASH diet emphasizes eating foods rich in fruits, vegetables, and low or non-fat dairy products to provide high intake of potassium as well as magnesium and calcium.[44] The results of these studies show that for anyone who is either hypertensive or at risk of developing high blood pressure they should consume adequate calcium, potassium, and magnesium on a daily basis.

When your diet lacks these minerals, supplementation may improve your blood pressure. If you eat plentiful amounts of vegetables, you are likely getting plenty of potassium. Potassium-rich foods include avocados, bananas, cantaloupe, honeydew melon, grapefruit, nectarines, oranges, asparagus, broccoli, cabbage, cauliflower, green peas, potatoes, and squash. Foods rich in magnesium include nuts, rice, bananas, potatoes, wheat germ, kidney and lima beans, soy, and molasses. Sufficient magnesium, on the other hand, is difficult to obtain through diet alone (see An Additional Note on Magnesium in the next subsection).

The DASH diet concluded that blood pressure could be reduced by an eating plan that is low in saturated fat, cholesterol, and total fat and high in fruits and vegetables, and low-fat dairy foods. On this note, I would agree with the notion of "high in fruits and vegetables", but would to take issue with the categorical "low in saturated fat, cholesterol and low-fat dairy foods." As I have analyzed above, cholesterol and saturated fats in and of themselves are not the culprits – the types of fats and what is happening along with the cholesterol (in terms of free radical activity) that are the most important issues to evaluate.

Of course, if it is inconvenient to purchase and prepare these fruits and vegetables, they are available in pill form. I had previously mentioned JuicePlus+ (www.juiceplus.com/+sk27973), which is a convenient, healthful way of getting plenty of these foods and minerals in pill form. Otherwise, there are plenty of quality supplements in the marketplace that offer these minerals straight in pill form as well.

An Additional Note on Magnesium

Magnesium may be the most important of the three valuable minerals noted above. Magnesium is required as a cofactor in hundreds of enzymatic processes within your cells. This wonderful mineral is a major factor in relaxing the smooth muscles within your blood vessels, thereby reducing blood pressure.[45] In addition, magnesium reduces your nerve and muscle excitability, stabilizes the conductivity of electrical impulses in your heart, and influences the proper transmission of chemicals in your body. Magnesium also controls circulating levels of norepinephrine and the synthesis of other blood pressure relieving chemicals in your body, called *serotonin* and *nitric oxide*.[46]

Recall the discussion previously regarding calcium channel blockers (prescription drugs) for blood pressure control. Remember how muscle cells in the arterioles can get excess calcium in the pores, which can cause a constriction of these blood vessels and that drugs called calcium channel blockers can block this excess calcium from constricting the blood vessels? Well, it just so happens that magnesium also directly offsets the constriction of blood vessels caused by calcium. Indeed, because of magnesium's primary role in this type of blood pressure regulation, scientists have called magnesium "nature's calcium channel blocker."

Sadly, drug companies cannot make money from a natural substance like magnesium, so they have developed a whole group of drugs called calcium channel blockers to do what magnesium does! In 2000, doctors wrote more than 95 million prescriptions for calcium blockers, including top sellers *amlo-dipine (Norvasc®), nifedipine (Procardia®), diltiazem (Cardizem®, Tiazac®)*, and others at a total cost of more than $4.5 billion. These drugs are not only costly, but they can also cause side effects as noted above (such as dizziness, palpitations, fatigue, tiredness, and swollen legs). Yet, many doctors do not hesitate to prescribe these drugs because they were never taught about magnesium.

Modern food production contributes to the problem by using inadequate amounts of magnesium in plant fertilizers, as well as by using accelerated growing techniques and different processing methods that reduce magnesium content. Today's dietary habits also exacerbate the problem. If you drink sodas and other popular beverages, the large amount of phosphates in these drinks interfere with your magnesium absorption. Further, if your diet contains large amounts of fat, salt, coffee, or alcohol this will interfere with your absorption of magnesium or you will just lose magnesium. If you take calcium supplements, you can increase this absorption and reduce your kidney's excretion of magnesium and other vital minerals. Because magnesium is not plentiful in foods, or at least the foods that you like to eat, magnesium supplementation may be effective in both preventing and controlling high blood pressure.

Despite all this, trying to determine if you have a magnesium deficiency is difficult. There is no simple, widely available test for magnesium deficiency. Mainstream medical laboratories measure your total serum (blood) magnesium. This measurement is not a very accurate identification of the problem because even if you are severely magnesium deficient, your body will maintain a normal blood level of magnesium by taking magnesium from your cells and bone. Therefore, a normal blood magnesium level can mask even a major magnesium deficiency.

Specialty laboratories can perform magnesium analyses on ionized blood, red blood cells, hair, and cells swabbed from the inner side of the cheek. These tests can be quite accurate and are frequently used by alternative doctors.

Now, those are the minerals that can address the issue of hypertension, There are a couple of well-known vitamins that are gaining notoriety as having a positive influence on blood pressure in addition to all of their many other benefits. The first one is Vitamin E.

Vitamins

Vitamin E

Vitamin E is an antioxidant derived from plants. This vitamin is part of a family of nutrients that includes two types of chemical substances, notably tocopherol and tocotrienols, each with their own subfamilies of alpha, beta, gamma and delta substances. Most commercial vitamin E supplements do not contain the gamma form of the vitamin, depriving you of the full range of its particular antioxidant effects. The vitamin E you buy at the local pharmacy is mostly alpha-tocopherol. Alpha-tocopherol is known to be an important antioxidant. But, when combined with other parts of the vitamin, the benefits are significantly enhanced. Tocotrienols have shown superior action in maintaining arterial health.[47] This wonder nutrient is so effective because it is a great scavenger of free radicals.[48]

Vitamin E supplements can help in the fight against hypertension. One manner in which vitamin E may control hypertension is through its actions as an antioxidant, molecules that decrease the destructive effects of our arch enemy, free radicals.[49] These highly reactive compounds, which as you learned above, are formed continuously in the body and are now being linked to a variety of disease states. But, these diseased states also include hypertension. Preliminary studie have shown that people who have hypertension often have low levels of essential antioxidants such as vitamin E.[50] Other studies with rats have shown that supplementation with a form of vitamin E (gamma tocotrienol) protected the animals against the development of age-related hypertension.[51]

Vitamin C

Like vitamin E, vitamin C is proving to be increasingly useful in treating more and more age-related disease states including heart disease, cancer and hypertension. Several studies have now shown that there is a significant link between vitamin C levels and hypertension. The lower the level of vitamin C, the higher the level of hypertension.[52]

What is adequate for blood pressure control? Well, most experts would conclude that at least 500 mg. of vitamin C daily would cause a significant drop in your blood pressure if you had hypertension. While some researchers believe that vitamin C controls hypertension through its antioxidant actions, others believe that vitamin C may also work through its role in modulating the activity of a chemically simple, yet very important gas known as nitric oxide.

Get more sunlight and UV light – and More Vitamin D

I went into great detail in Part I on the benefits of sunlight on palpitations. As I noted in Part I, exposure to sunlight can actually significantly lower your blood pressure. In fact, several studies have suggested that the further from the equator you move, the more risk there is of high blood pressure. Conversely, the farther one gets from the equator, the more likely you are to find people with high blood pressure. Lack of exposure to ultraviolet light may actually contribute to the rise in blood pressure in higher latitudes. And the theory may explain why Afro-Americans and black people in Europe have a greater risk of high blood pressure than Caucasians in those countries or blacks who live in Africa.

Since sunlight plays an important role in your synthesis of vitamin D, the farther away from the equator you are, the less ultraviolet exposure and the less vitamin D that is synthesized in your body. And, the greater amount of pigment in your skin, such as heavily tanned people or blacks, require six times the amount of ultraviolet B (UVB) light to produce the same amount of vitamin D found in lighter-skinned people. While 20% to 30% of UVB radiation is transmitted through white skin, only 5% is transmitted through deeply pigmented skin.

This is yet another significant bit of information that clearly goes against the grain of the recommendations most of us receive to avoid any sun exposure. On the contrary, we all need sunlight to stay healthy.

Researchers theorize that UV exposure leads to the release of chemicals in the brain called endorphins, which are linked to both pain relief and euphoric feelings. UV exposure from sun tanning beds leads to pain relief and euphoric feelings.[53] Researchers believe that decreased vitamin D production actually results in the increased production of a certain hormone that actually serves to increase blood pressure. Other studies have actually found that vitamin D tends to suppress the *renin-angiotensin* system we discussed above and this serves to lower blood pressure (Hobday).

The advice of the traditional medical community to stay out of the sun, because it will cause cancer, may actually be one of the major reasons why there is actually an increase in heart disease! You and everyone else need sunlight and when you don't receive it, your health may decline. You just need to exert common sense guidelines and always avoid getting sun burned. You should probably limit exposure during the peak hours of the day. However, an hour a day of sunshine is important to maintain optimal health.

In addition to vitamins and minerals dealing with the issue of high blood pressure, certain amino acids have shown to similarly have a very positive effect as well.

Amino Acids

Arginine and Nitric Oxide

Arginine is an amino acid and is an excellent weapon in the fight against hypertension. Arginine works through its ability to produce a simple gas made up of nitrogen and oxygen (called "nitric oxide" (NO)), that penetrates and crosses the membranes of almost all cells in the human body and helps regulate many cellular functions. Remember our earlier reference to endothelial cells? They are the ones that line the inside of blood vessels. Well, NO is extremely important because it regulates the tone of these endothelial cells, causing them to become smoother and softer. For your body to maintain a healthy circulatory system, it must produce healthy amounts of NO. So, when your body is producing adequate amounts of NO, plaque formation and blood clots are less likely to occur (because the NO interferes with the coagulation of blood platelets, those small disk-shaped bodies made up of cell fragments that are responsible for clotting). As I noted above, if they (the endothelial cells) become dysfunctional, they can cause spasms or constrictions of the blood vessels that can then lead to hypertension. Studies bear out the conclusion that there can be significant decreases in blood pressure taking arginine supplements.

In this connection, Nobel Prize winning author Louis Ignarro considers NO as your body's "natural cardiovascular wonder drug" and notes in his best selling book, *NO More Heart Disease*, that NO relaxes and enlarges the blood vessels, making sure that blood can nourish the heart. He further states that "NO influences the functioning of virtually every bodily organ, including the lungs, liver, kidneys, stomach, genitals, and, of course, the heart" and "the difference between health and illness is often a function of the level of NO activity in your body." Interestingly, this is just another example of natural strategies not only being essentially devoid of negative side effects, but also actually having positive ones, like increased libido and sexual stamina associated with nitric oxide.

So, I have discussed vitamins, minerals and amino acids in connection with improvement in blood pressure. A discussion of this topic would not be complete without the role that the essential fatty acids play in controlling blood pressure.

Essential Fatty Acids

Fish oil

Once again fish oil "takes the limelight." Fish oil supplements containing the omega-3 fatty acids EPA and DHA, in addition to the many other host of benefits discussed above, are also effective in controlling hypertension. Fish oil is one of the few supplements, sometimes otherwise referred to as "nutriceuticals" that has been endorsed by a major health organization in the United States – in this case, the American Heart Association (AHA). Studies have shown that fish oil supplements, besides decreasing triglycerides and LDL cholesterol levels, cause a statistically significant decrease in both systolic and diastolic blood pressure measurements.

Herbs

Garlic

And, don't forget about herbs. Garlic has long been known for its cardiovascular benefits, including the lowering of blood pressure.[54] As an added feature, it can also lower cholesterol (see the discussion on garlic in Chapter 11 on cholesterol), reduce triglyceride levels, discourage clot formation, and promote blood circulation. A typical dose of garlic is 900 mg of garlic powder per day, standardized to contain 1.3% allicin. This provides about 12,000 mcg. (micrograms) of allicin per day. This dosage is also recommended for lowering high cholesterol.

Garlic can also thin the blood. But, it should not be combined with prescription blood-thinners such as *Coumadin* (*warfarin*) or *Trental* (*pentoxifylline*) or with natural blood-thinners such as vitamin E or ginkgo. It is usually recommended that people taking garlic stop in the weeks before and after any type of surgery.

Sadly, I am not very high on garlic because garlic has been a sensitivity for me in terms of being a catalyst for heart arrhythmias.

Hawthorn

Another herb that impacts your blood pressure is hawthorn. Hawthorn is a very well known heart tonic in traditional herbal medicine. It has been used in Europe and China for centuries as a folk remedy. It is believed to decrease blood pressure, increase heart muscle contraction, increase blood flow to the heart muscle, and decrease heart rate.

So far I have pointed out vitamins, minerals, amino acids, fatty acids and herbs. But, certain enzymes play a part in regulating blood pressure as well.

Enzymes

Coenzyme Q10

Once again, our friend, CoQ10 shows up. If you recall, CoQ10 is a compound found naturally in the energy-producing center of the cell known as the mitochondria. CoQ10 is involved in the making of an important molecule known as ATP. ATP serves as your cell's major energy source and drives a number of biological processes including muscle contraction and the production of protein. A good analogy for CoQ10's role is similar to the role of a spark plug in a car engine. Just as the car cannot function without that initial spark, the human body cannot function without CoQ10. CoQ10 also works as an antioxidant.

CoQ10 deficiency has been shown to be present in many people (as much as 39%) with high blood pressure. This finding alone suggests a need for CoQ10 supplementation. However, CoQ10 appears to provide benefits beyond correction of any deficiency. In several studies CoQ10 has actually been shown to lower blood pressure in people with hypertension.[55] The effect of CoQ10 on blood pressure is usually not seen until after 4-12 weeks of therapy. Typical reductions in both systolic and diastolic blood pressure with CoQ10 therapy in patients with high blood pressure are in the 10% range.

An eight-week trial completed in 1999 certainly adds evidence to support the use of CoQ10 in hypertension and may provide a better understanding of its action. In this trial, conducted at the Centre of Nutrition at the Medical Hospital and Research Centre in India, 59 men with hypertension were randomized to receive 120 mg per day CoQ10 or placebo. Both systolic and diastolic pressure decreased significantly in the CoQ10 group – an average of 16 and 9 points, respectively. The researchers also measured glucose and insulin levels and saw significant decreases in those, as well. There is increasing evidence that as many as 50 percent of individuals with hypertension may also be insulin resistant. When insulin is not working effectively, your body produces more, which leads to higher blood pressure. This trial suggests Coenzyme Q10 may improve the way insulin works and, as a beneficial side effect, lower blood pressure.

At any rate, there are scores of studies that support the conclusion that CoQ10 demonstrably helps with diastolic and systolic pressure, plain and simple.

Hormones

Melatonin

This discussion would not be complete without addressing certain hormones that positively impact your blood pressure.

Heart attacks most often occur when blood flow is most constricted, which is early in the morning. This is also when levels of the sleep hormone melatonin drop quite a bit and the levels of the stress hormone cortisol increase.

Melatonin interacts with blood vessels through receptor sites on the coronary arteries. Taking melatonin before bedtime may decrease your blood pressure as much as if you were taking an anti-hypertensive drug. While melatonin also tends to increase the quality and quantity of sleep, in some people it does the opposite. Many people report that it may put you to sleep, but staying asleep is sometimes a problem.

Certain Foods and Drinks

Pomegranates

There are other foods and drinks that impact blood pressure. Surprisingly, pomegranates may also be of benefit in reducing the harsh consequences of hypertension.[56]

In an Israeli study, systolic blood pressure was reduced by 21% after one year of pomegranate juice consumption. This effect is believed to be related to the particularly potent antioxidant properties of the pomegranate. Other studies confirmed the effectiveness of the pomegranate in lowering blood pressure.[57]

Tea, Not Coffee

There is some evidence to support the conclusion that high amounts of coffee can trigger irregular heartbeats and can increase your homocysteine levels (if you recall higher than normal homocysteine levels can indicate damaged blood vessels). What is considered to be high is difficult to determine, although more than two cups a day would normally be deemed excessive.

Tea is the second most consumed beverage in the world, second only to water. A recently published research study revealed that habitual tea drinkers may significantly reduce their risk of hypertension.[58] In fact, however, habitual tea drinkers who ingested 120-599 mL of tea daily exhibited a 46% reduction in hypertension compared to non-habitual drinkers. Even more striking was the 65% reduction in hypertension in those who ingested over 600 mL of tea daily compared to non-habitual drinkers.

Green tea would have the added advantages of mildly lowering LDL cholesterol and increasing HDL cholesterol, reducing atherosclerosis, and having antioxidant properties. However, while tea would be a safe as well as reasonably reliable strategy to reduce high blood pressure, there is evidence that green tea can cause arrhythmias in some people, including yours truly. Thus, if you are prone to irregular heartbeats, then your best bet is to drink decaffeinated tea but stay away from green tea.

The Natural Blood Pressure Solution II – What You Should Not Do

Do Not Continue to Eat Like You Do

I know, you are saying that this is easier said than done. But, extra pounds mean extra work for the heart, which must exert additional pressure to push the blood through the extra mile of blood vessels that come with each pound of excess fat. Obesity is literally a huge public health problem in America, in particular and is a major contributor to many modern diseases, including hypertension. Being obese puts you at increased risk of developing hypertension at an early age, as well as developing more severe hypertension. However, with weight loss, hypertension can be significantly controlled.

Recognizing, of course, that I am not here to write a book on weight loss techniques, as there are thousands of theories, plans, systems, pills, strategies, and the like to help you lose those extra pounds. But, there are some very basic steps that can be readily and quickly implemented very inexpensively to curb your appetite and to cause you to shed pounds.

Avoid Processed Sugar

Significantly reduce your intake of processed sugars, whether it is white table sugar, high fructose corn syrup, fructose, glucose, or whatever. Try to stay as far away as you can. One of these days you will eventually realize that processed sugar is probably the most toxic substance consumed by mankind on a regular basis. In fact, the only thing that may be worse may be pure poison. Sadly, your mind and your body have been programmed by big business into believing that this substance is an acceptable foodstuff. Your body has been lured by the façade of provocative advertising and the irresistible temptation of instant gratification, all the while being succumbed to the highly addictive properties of this most dangerous substance.

Indeed, according to Dr. Joseph Mercola, in his book "*The No Grain Diet*", sugar is one of the biggest enemies that you will face in your pursuit of a healthy eating program and a program that will lower your blood pressure. Sugar appears in almost everything you eat and drink, making it virtually impossible to avoid. There is no doubt that sugar increases your insulin levels, which can lead to high blood pressure, high cholesterol, heart disease, diabetes, weight gain, premature aging and many more negative side effects. Controlling insulin levels is one of the most important things you can do to optimize your health, and avoiding sugar is essential to do this.

Sugars also mess up the proper regulation of fluid and hormonal levels in your body. Sugar has the potential of inducing abnormal metabolic processes if you are a normal healthy individual and to promote chronic degenerative diseases. Sugar can cause less effective functioning of two blood proteins that you have (albumin, and lipoproteins), which may reduce your body's ability to handle fat and cholesterol. Sugar can cause hormonal imbalance (some hormones become under-active and others become overactive). This is why sugar can even exacerbate your PMS (if your are female) and even cause epileptic seizures.

And, did you ever wonder why you tend to get sick more often than you would like? Just think how many sweets you eat, sodas you consume, and cereals you crunch down. Sugar suppresses your immune system and weakens your defenses against bacterial infection. Sugar upsets the vitamin and mineral relationships in your body (e.g., causes a deficiency in chromium and interferes with the absorption of important vitamins and minerals such as Vitamin E, calcium and magnesium). This leads to sickness and disease – sometimes chronic. There are studies that show that excess sugar can lead to various cancers, such as prostate, breast, gallbladder, ovarian and rectal. Hypoglycemia, Crohn's disease, Alzheimer's disease, ulcerative colitis, arthritis, asthma and osteoporosis are further illnesses linked to excessive, and sometimes even minimal, sugar consumption. Sugar can cause yeast infections, gallstones, and even multiple sclerosis. And, if you think emphysema is just limited to smokers, guess again – sugar can actually cause this irreversible and incurable disease. High sucrose intake can even be an important risk factor in lung cancer.

Do you have kids? Are they often hyperactive, anxious and cranky? Can't figure out why? Well, you should know that sugars cause a rapid rise in adrenaline levels. Sugar can also worsen the symptoms of your children if they have attention deficit hyperactivity disorder (ADHD). This can result in adversely affecting their grades and cause numerous learning disorders. Then, just take away their candy bars, cake, doughnuts, and soda for a while. You just may find that they will concentrate better, have better grades and be much, much calmer. One study reports that in juvenile rehabilitation camps, when children were put on a low sugar diet, there was a 44% drop in antisocial behavior.

And, you know that phrase, "stunting your growth"? Sugar is probably the number one culprit in connection with this problem, since it clearly causes a decrease in growth hormone. High sugar consumption can lead to substantial decrease in gestation duration among adolescents. It also can make your skin age by changing the structure of collagen. Interestingly, sugar increases estradiol (the most potent form of naturally occurring estrogen) in men. Do you know that if you are male and in your upper 50's or older, sugar consumption you may actually cause you to have more estrogen than testosterone? In other words, sugar gets you older faster!

Also, have you had a physical lately? Did you have blood work that showed elevated triglyceride levels and low HDLs (the good cholesterol)? Well, instead of getting a script for some ridiculously expensive, sometimes addictive, drug that has 25 possible negative side effects, consider your diet. Sugar has been known to cause a marked increase in triglyceride levels, the increase in LDLs (the bad cholesterol) and the lowering of HDLs. Sugar is even the catalyst for atherosclerosis.

Yes, sugar tastes good, but what does it do for you other than give you tooth decay, periodontal disease and an acidic and frequently painful digestive tract. Indeed, sugar even increases the risk of gastric cancer. It also combines and destroys phosphatase, an enzyme that makes the process of digestion more difficult.

Other key organs can also be devastated by sugar. Examples include the causation of cataracts and nearsightedness in connection with your eyesight. Sugar can wreak havoc on your liver, pancreas and kidneys in that it can cause these organs to become uncharacteristically enlarged. In the kidneys, sugar can be a contributor towards kidney stones. And, in the elderly, sugar is one of the key problems with respect to regular and effective bowel movements.

Sugar will make your joints ache and your tendons more brittle. Further, it causes a loss of tissue elasticity and function; that is, the more sugar you eat the more elasticity and function you lose. Sugar has a history of causing gout, which is an inflammatory disease of your joints.

Hopefully, after all that you are ready to say "Ok, I surrender, I have heard enough." Hopefully, you have and you will do something about it. Suffice it to say, sugar may be the most toxic substance known to mankind that is consumed in large quantities and is legal, including cigarettes!

Avoid Late Night Sweet Snacks

There are just a few points to remember here for a quick weight loss fix. That is, simply severely restrict your intake of food after your dinner meal. You'll be amazed how much weight you will lose with this little tip. In fact, eat dinner as early as possible. The problem, however, with this latter idea is that you will more likely get hungry the earlier you eat. If you must eat something later in the evening, restrict your eating to protein foods such as a piece of chicken or some nuts. The protein group of foods should not cause the gaining of weight. Also, the nuts will provide some of the good fats, so that your craving for food will subside.

Having said all that, you are probably saying that you sometimes crave something sweet. To begin with, the above discussion on sugar should dissuade you from consuming any significant amount of sugary items. But, if you still cannot resist, conduct the following experiment to prove that your desire to eat sugary carbohydrates, like cake, cookies, ice cream and other "desserts" is largely the result of a distorted combination of a psychological craving for sweets and a biological craving for wholesome foods. So, take some protein food, like chicken as noted above and also even consume a few nuts, like almonds or cashews. Then, have whatever sweet item you are craving. But, just chew up the sweet item and experience whatever taste satisfaction you seem to be craving, but before swallowing, spit the chewed up dessert or sweet snack out into the kitchen sink and maybe wash your mouth out with water (but make sure you do not swallow any of the sweet item). Recognizing, of course, that this is an experiment (and hopefully you are not doing this in front of mixed company or really anyone for that matter), experience how you feel, which is probably quite fulfilled. This simply proves that you are not consuming the sweets for any nutritional purpose, and there is absolutely no reason to ingest the sweet item. Sugary carbohydrates just give you greater instantaneous pleasure that you typically mistake for wholesome food that your body really is craving.

Hopefully, this experiment will further motivate you to get off the sugar and on to more nutritional foods and less pounds to carry around.

So, you might say, "I need to have some sweet things. Isn't there any alternative to sugar in the traditional sense?" Well, the good news is that there is an alternative. Consider the following.

As an Alternative, Use Natural and Nutritious Sugar Substitutes

What many people don't realize about artificial sweeteners is that they don't help you lose weight! They actually feed or catalyze your sweet tooth, making you crave more sugar rather than less. There is also evidence that they slow down digestion and increase appetite.

Keep in mind that we are not talking about using saccharin and aspartame (under the brands *Equal* or *Nutrasweet*). Nor are we talking about *Sucralose*, which is found in many sweeteners, including *Splenda*, which has been linked to accelerating or causing migraines, mood and sleep disturbances, dizziness, fuzzy thinking, and an inability to concentrate.[59]

Aspartame, found in *Nutrasweet* and *Equal* can create an undesirable stimulation of the brain in less than positive ways, and can also lead to neurological and endocrine problems and can even be addictive. Aspartame sweeteners have generated more complaints to the FDA of adverse reactions than any non-drug. In fact, more than 75% of all non-drug complaints to the FDA are about aspartame. These complaints include headaches, dizziness, mood changed, numbness, vomiting or nausea, muscle cramps and spasms, and abdominal pain and cramps. There are also sizable numbers reporting vision changes, joint pains, skin lesions, memory loss, and seizures. This is only a small fraction of the actual adverse reactions caused by aspartame. Most people would not associate the problem with aspartame, and even if they did, only a small fraction of people or doctors would take the time to report it to the FDA. Doctors estimate that for every reported adverse reaction, 10 to 100 go unrecognized or unreported.[60]

As reported by the Conference of the American College of Physicians and leading physicians and scientists appearing before the U.S. Congress, the excitatory characteristics of aspartame could lower the threshold for, and even cause, seizures, mania, depression, or other psychological or central nervous system disorders. These brain/mood symptoms brought on by aspartame could easily be caused by the changes in brain chemistry triggered by elevations of an amino acid called *"phenylalanine"*. While there have been numerous studies showing aspartame's safety, the problem with these studies is that they used aspartame capsules rather than the commonly used form of aspartame mixed and stored in food.

Even more significant, perhaps, is the role of methanol or methyl alcohol (also called "wood alcohol"), which makes up 10% of aspartame. The methanol is further broken down into, believe it or not, formaldehyde (a known carcinogen), formic acid (a poison excreted by ants) and diketopiperazine (DKP, which studies have shown to cause brain tumors).[61] Absorption of methanol is hastened if aspartame has broken down, as it does when it is heated, used in hot drinks or decomposed during prolonged storage. So, if you don't do anything, don't use aspartame in your hot drinks, such as tea or coffee. Methanol is specifically toxic to the optic nerve and potentially can cause blindness. The poisoning effects of taking methanol are cumulative.

Anecdotally, the Center for Behavioral Medicine, Professor of Clinical Psychiatry, Northeastern Ohio Universities College of Medicine analyzed 164 studies which were felt to have relevance to human safety questions. Of those studies, 74 studies had aspartame industry-related sponsorship and 90 were funded without any industry money. Of the 90 non-industry-sponsored studies, 83 (92%) identified one or more problems with aspartame. Of the 7 studies that did not find a problem, 6 of those studies were conducted by the FDA. Given that a number of FDA officials went to work for the aspartame industry immediately following approval (including the former FDA Commissioner), many consider these studies to be equivalent to industry-sponsored research. Of the 74 aspartame industry-sponsored studies, all 74 (100%) claimed that no problems were found with aspartame.

Stevia to the Rescue

There are only two sweeteners worth mentioning in the same breath as the word "healthy." The first is called "*stevia.*" Stevia is an herb that has been used as a sweetener in South America for hundreds of years. It is calorie-free, and the powdered concentrate is 300 times sweeter than sugar. Because the human body does not metabolize the chemical in stevia (called "sweet glycosides") (as they pass right through the normal elimination channels) your body obtains no calories from stevia. Whether the stevia products are called stevia, stevioside, rebaudioside, stevia extract, or stevia concentrate, if they are in their pure unadulterated form, they do not adversely affect blood glucose levels and may be used freely by both diabetics and hypoglycemics. For people with blood pressure or weight problems, stevia is a most desirable sweetener.

In all of its current forms stevia has a taste unique to itself. Along with its sweetness there is also a bitter component. The poorer the quality of the leaf the more bitterness is evident in the taste. In good consumer products, however, this bitter flavor disappears as does the slight licorice taste of whole-leaf products when appropriately diluted for consumption. Unlike artificial sweeteners, the sweet glycosides do not break down in heat, which makes stevia an excellent sweetener for cooking and baking. However, having stated that, my experience is that many of the packaged, powdered stevia products that you get in progressive grocery stores and health food stores are not meant for cooking and baking, does break down and in fact does not retain its sweetness. So, exercise some care in choosing your stevia product if you intend to use it for cooking and baking.

Stevia is also one of the most health restoring plants on earth. What stevia does both inside the body and on the skin is rather fascinating. Native to Paraguay, it is a small green plant bearing leaves, which have a delicious and refreshing taste. Besides the intensely sweet glycosides (a glycoside is any of a group of organic compounds, occurring abundantly in plants, that yield a sugar and one or more non-sugar substances on hydrolysis, such as *steviosides, rebaudiosides* and *dulcosides*), various studies have found the leaf to contain proteins, fiber, carbohydrates, iron, phosphorus, calcium, potassium, sodium, magnesium, zinc, rutin (a flavonoid), true vitamin A, vitamin C and an oil which contains 53 other constituents. Quality stevia leaves and whole leaf concentrate are nutritious, natural dietary supplements offering numerous health benefits.

Stevia is widely used all over the world. In Japan, for example, it claims 41% of the sweetener market, including sugar, and was used in Japanese Diet Coke until the company replaced it with aspartame to "standardize" worldwide. There have not been any reports of toxicity with stevia, which is consumed by millions of people daily.

As a dietary supplement, scientific research has indicated that stevia effectively regulates blood sugar and brings it toward a normal balance. Stevia is sold in some South American countries as an aid to people with diabetes and hypoglycemia. Since its introduction into the U.S., numerous people have reported that taking 20-30 drops with each meal brought their blood glucose levels to normal or near normal within a short time period. Obviously each individual's condition is different and such experimentation should be done under the supervision of a qualified physician. An important benefit for hypo-glycemics is stevia's tonic action, which enhances increased energy levels and mental acuity.

Studies have also indicated that stevia tends to lower elevated blood pressure but does not seem to affect normal blood pressure. Stevia also inhibits the growth and reproduction of some bacteria and other infectious organisms, including the bacteria that cause tooth decay and gum disease. This may help explain why users of stevia enhanced products report a lower incidence of colds and flu and why it has such exceptional qualities when used as a mouthwash or added to toothpaste.

An Alternative to Stevia – TheraSweet™

Another sweetener worthy of mention is a blend of substances called TheraSweet™ formulated by a company called Living Fuel located in Florida. TheraSweet™ was designed to be a safe and healthy alternative to the artificial sweeteners on the market today. TheraSweet™ tastes and looks like sugar, but without any of the bitter aftertaste of conventional sweeteners. And, unlike other artificial sweeteners, it is completely natural. Xylitol is the essential ingredient in TheraSweet™. Xyliltol is obtained from organic sources, such as fruits, vegetables, and hardwood trees. Tagatose, the second largest ingredient in TheraSweet™, is derived from natural sources as well – yogurt, cheeses and fruit. But, besides being used as a sweetener, TheraSweet™ also contains other therapeutic, health-promoting benefits.

Xylitol has a small glycemic index, but it is still 20 times less than sugar. It is being used all over the world as a safe choice for diabetics. Tagatose is a low-calorie sweetener, which, unlike most substitute sweeteners, withstands the heat of baking without breaking down, and it browns like sugar. They have also included probiotics, which help the body by synthesizing enzymes that increase the digestibility of protein, improve bowel function, modulating the immune system, increasing the production of antibodies, amongst many other benefits.

On top of all that they added glycine, an amino acid found in the protein of all life forms. Glycine is required for the maintenance of the central nervous system and is an important neuroinhibitor (brain relaxant). Glycine also plays an important role in the immune system, where it is used in the synthesis of other non-essential amino acids. Glycine is also a constituent of a vital bile acid, and together with cysteine and glutamic acid, makes up glutathione – a major liver detoxifier and a destroyer of free-radicals.

Eliminate White Bread and Grain Products

There is another "don't do" in your quest to fight high blood pressure. This might sound difficult and if you love to eat breads, pasta, cereal, pastries and muffins, it's time to re-think this eating practice. Any meal or snack high in carbohydrates (and those items epitomize the terms "high in carbohydrates") generates a rapid rise in blood glucose. To adjust for this rise, your pancreas secretes the hormone insulin into your bloodstream, which lowers your glucose levels. Insulin is, though, essentially a storage hormone, evolved over those millions of years of humans prior to the agricultural age, to store the excess calories from carbohydrates in the form of fat in case of famine. Insulin, stimulated by these excess carbohydrates in your overabundant consumption of grains and starches (not to mention sugary items), is responsible for your bulging stomachs and fat rolls on your thighs and chins.

Even worse, high insulin levels suppress two other important hormones, called "*glucagons*" and "*growth hormones.*" They are responsible for burning your fat and sugar and promoting your muscle development, respectively. So insulin from excess carbohydrates promotes fat in your body, and then wards off your body's ability to lose that fat.

Do Not Continue to Consume Excessive Salt

This step should be part of a weight reduction program as well as a general heart health program even if you are not overweight. Generally, salt (sodium chloride) is a chemical that is needed by your body in that salt regulates the fluid balance of your cells and plasma. Too little salt will cause you to become dehydrated because you cannot retain water. However, if you consume too much salt, high blood pressure results (falling short of the conclusion that salt actually causes high blood pressure). Salt restriction should be a major part of your new "program." Limit your salt intake to less than 2,400 mg (about one teaspoon) a day (keep in mind that the average American consumes between 9,000 and 12,000 mg per day)!

Lowering your salt intake is a daunting task since the average American is increasingly eating in restaurants or eating processed or prepared foods, not to mention salt being used as a natural preservative for meats and vegetables.

The best place to start a salt reduction program is to check the nutritional labels on the foods you eat. You will be quite surprised as to high salt content in most foods. When you are in a restaurant ask for light or, ideally, no salt on foods.

Additionally, consider using reduced or no-salt packaged products. Take the saltshaker away from your table top and substitute it with an herbal mixture. Try to cut down on processed, canned or convenience foods (like frozen dinners, which are easy but dangerous). Also, avoid soy sauce, teriyaki sauce as they are very high in sodium. And, cut down on your use of cured foods (like bacon) and foods packaged in brine, like pickles. Limit your use of mustard, ketchup and other condiments. Replace the salt in your food preparation with lemon juice, orange juice, vinegar and/or herbs.

The above protocol may be hard at first, but after a while, foods will taste salty enough with the little salt that you use. Then, after a while, when you eat foods that have an average amount of salt, they will taste excessively salty and you will be surprised that you ever withstood foods with salt levels that most foods contain.

Summary on Losing Weight and Fat

So, losing weight and fat is quite simple. You don't have take spend a fortune on pills, exercise equipment or diet programs. You can easily lose 10-20% of your body weight by avoiding sugars, white flours and grains, reducing your salt and don't eat a late dinner. And, above all, don't eat carbohydrates after dinner. Exercise is great and definitely important to your heart health and weight loss regimen, but adhere to those eating prohibitions and you will be shocked how much better you look and feel.

Do Not Continue to Smoke if You are a Smoker

You should not be surprised to learn that cigarette use is a major contributing factor of high blood pressure, not to mention other forms of heart disease. In fact, several experts in the field rank smoking to be the top risk factor for cardiovascular disease. Even just smoking one cigarette can cause your transient blood pressure increases of 10 points or more. If you smoke on a regular basis you will have a sustained rise in your blood pressure due to the effects of nicotine and other dangerous chemicals found in cigarettes.

Although nicotine is the primary agent in cigarettes that everyone focuses on, there are other chemicals and compounds that are just as bad, like tar and carbon monoxide. These chemicals lead to the development and build-up of fatty plaque in your arteries by primarily injuring your blood vessel walls. They also negatively impact cholesterol and fibrin, the blood clotting material you don't want too much of at the wrong time.

Here are some other interesting facts that you should know about before you light up again. If you smoke, your chance of dying of cardiovascular disease is about twice as much as a non-smoker, and as far as dying suddenly from heart problems, smoking is the leading cause. In other words, smokers who have heart attacks are more likely to die and die suddenly (within an hour) than are non-smokers. And, for those who are exposed to secondhand smoke at work or at home, your chances are increased 30% of having cardiovascular disease. And, this does not include the risk of other diseases, such as lung cancer. Indeed, there is excess of an 80% chance that you will ultimately die within 5 years from lung cancer – if you live long enough to get the disease!

And, if you are a woman, it gets even scarier. Smoking reduces the protective nature of your estrogen. Studies have shown that if you smoke, you are 39 times more likely to have a heart attack and 22 times more likely to have stroke than any one else who does not smoke!

Last but certainly not least, as noted in the Chapter 4 above on causation of irregular heartbeats, addictive substances such as cigarette smoking can provoke arrhythmias.

Want another interesting fact about smoking, in fact, an amazing, shocking fact? Despite all these horrible things about smoking tobacco, cigarettes are the only product in this country where the ingredients do not need to be listed! Surprised? Well, maybe you should ponder if it is remotely possible that the tobacco industry makes a few dollars of contributions to the campaigns of our politicians, who in turn dictate to the FDA?

But, the good news for smokers is that there is reason and motivation to stop now, notably, that a smoker's risk of a heart attack is cut in half after only one year without smoking. With all the other known health risks associated with smoking-heart disease, diabetes and impotence, to name just a few, smoking cessation should be at the top of anyone's list that is looking to improve his or her blood pressure and overall health.

It is basic human nature to promptly respond to an immediate threat to your health and safety. Unfortunately, if you are like most people, you will wait until there is some pain or discomfort before you respond in some fashion. Until that time, you typically have other things more pressing to worry about or you rationalize with an attitude of "it cannot happen to me." In chapter 10, you learned that threats such as hypertension can take years or decades to exert its damaging effects on the body, and sometimes it is too late to correct it effectively and completely. Such an unconcerned attitude can readily lead to heart disease, not to mention other diseases and an early death. By following a healthy lifestyle that includes a diet high in fruits and vegetables, avoiding all tobacco products and as many foods as possible that contain processed sugars, getting a reasonable amount of sunshine, maintaining a reasonable weight and taking safe and effective supplements, crippling diseases such as hypertension can be prevented from destroying your health and taking your life – without prescription drugs!

Yes, high blood pressure is a real killer, and even more destructive than high cholesterol. Do not wait for your doctor's instruction. You can start taking steps to prevent hypertension today – naturally and safely.

Some Final Thoughts

"Our health always seems much more valuable after we lose it."

—Author Unknown

Palpitations are a symptom described as the sensation of having an irregular heartbeat. These are sometimes also known as arrhythmias. This is a fairly common symptom that just about everyone experiences at one time or another. Palpitations occur when the heart beats irregularly. Whether or not palpitations are of medical concern is ultimately determined by medical history, physical exam findings, and testing. You should know when it's time to go to see your physician because the palpitations have become sustained and very uncomfortable, or they are associated with another symptom such as shortness of breath. Until that time, there are non-drug measures that you can take to control, alleviate and/or even eliminate the symptoms.

Heart rhythm is controlled by factors directly related as well as completely unrelated to the operation of the heart itself. The most common damage to the heart's "wiring" comes from damage caused by decreased blood flow from clogged coronary arteries, or from muscle death caused by a heart attack. Additionally, just as certain drugs and toxins can affect heart rhythm, foods, food additives and beverages such as caffeine (as well as other stimulants), alcohol, and dairy can trigger arrhythmias as well.

Yet, the heart has an amazing ability to tolerate markedly abnormal rhythms. If you experience sustained palpitations for the first time you should see a physician before taking any medications or special nutrients to determine the nature of the problem – whether it represents a serious heart abnormality or a benign arrhythmia. No matter what the cause of an irregular heartbeat, always ensuring that the heart gets enough blood is essential.

Unfortunately, the majority of anti-arrhythmic drugs have pro-arrhythmic effects. That is to say, they can themselves cause arrhythmias. Invasive strategies are risky and not fool-proof. The medical profession admits its shortcomings when it comes to the prevention, treatment and cure of nuisance and otherwise non-life threatening rhythms such as PVCs, PACs and AFIB (unaccompanied by other heart disease). There are, however, a number of safe, natural strategies you can use to prevent, suppress and/or beat these arrhythmias without drugs, without surgery, without invasive surgery and without negative side effects.

Your heart is considered to be the most important organ in your body. Don't take your heart for granted. Treat it like a trusted, hard-working life-long friend that every minute of every day puts its life on the line for you. Certainly from a financial standpoint, with healthcare costs rising at unprecedented levels coupled with a very shaky Medicare system (from a financial standpoint), you simply cannot afford to risk contracting any form of heart disease – literally.

No one can really look out for your best interests other than you, so be proactive and follow the many steps to curb arrhythmias and stem heart disease as outlined in this book. You will reap the rewards of living your life the way you want to – on your own terms, healthfully and happily and with peace of mind.

Stuart B. Kalb, Juris Doctor (J.D.)

Stuart B. Kalb is a presently an estate, elder law and retirement planning attorney and is a principal in the Law Offices of Kalb & Abelbeck, P.C., Dallas, Texas. Mr. Kalb has over 30 years extensive experience in creating numerous state-of-the-art retirement, estate, business succession and asset preservation plans. His additional areas of concentration include asset protection for the elderly and bio-ethics.

Mr. Kalb's unique services not only include protecting the wealth of his clients, but also include something very special – protecting the health of his clients as well as his friends and relatives. He is presently the owner and operator of Life-style Enhancement Enterprises, LLC, a company that specializes in natural, organic and safe nutritional products, and particularly products that focus on preventative heart health. He is presently writing two books – *Keeping Your Mind Sharp at Any Age,* which discusses seven natural and safe ways to prevent Alzheimer's disease and other forms of dementia – without drugs, surgery or invasive procedures and *Never Grow Old: Aging Healthfully Into Your Hundreds and Beyond.*

He has co-authored the books, *"Legacy: Plan, Protect and Preserve Your Estate", "Ways and Means – How to Protect Your Retirement Savings", "Generations – Planning Your Legacy".* Mr. Kalb is also a founding member of the National Association of Retirement and Wealth Preservation Advisors.

Formerly, Mr. Kalb was a healthcare attorney and represented hospitals in connection with various legal matters. He was also a Senior Tax Attorney for the United States Treasury Department. In this role, he was responsible for handling litigation in United States Tax Court and has represented the Commissioner of Internal Revenue in approximately thirty (30) trials. In addition, he has handled hundreds of Tax Court cases that were disposed of through settlement or other means. Mr. Kalb also served as Regional Tax Shelter Coordinator and Assistant Director, Southeast Region Tax Shelter Program (Office of Chief Counsel, U.S. Treasury Dept.). In this capacity, he handled the tax litigation and tax controversies with respect to large dollar volume cases as well as raising significant and complex issues. He also acted as consultant to Government Accounting Office regarding present and future status of tax shelter activity in the United States.

He is licensed to practice in all courts in the states of Texas and Florida, the U.S. Supreme Court, the U.S. Tax Court, the U.S. Circuit Court of Appeals (5th Circuit), the U.S. Federal District Court, and the U.S. Claims Court.

He received his bachelor's and law degree (Juris Doctor) from the University of Florida and has also received a master of laws degree in taxation (LL.M Taxation) from that university. His law review article appeared in the University of Florida Law Review entitled "The Deductibility of Post-Graduate Legal Education Expenses" (Summer 1975).

Mr. Kalb lives in Plano, Texas and is married with two grown children and one grandchild. When time permits, he enjoys golf, tennis, racquetball, weight training, billiards, table tennis, bowling, football, and softball.

Additional References

1. Jourven, et al., *Heart-Rate Profel During Exercise as a Predictor of Sudden Death*, N Engl. J Med. 2005; 352;1951-8; J. Intern. Med. 2000; 247: 231-2392005

2. American Journal of Clinical Nutrition, Vol.77, No. 3, 532-54 March 2003

3. According to Circulation: Journal of the American Heart Association, June 3, 2003; Dr. Hal Huggins, D.D.S., M.S., who is considered to be one of the best authorities on the mercury issue; and, the Foundation For Toxic-Free Dentistry

4. See Mercola and Klinghardt, *Mercury Toxicity and Systemic Elimination Agents*

5. O'Keefe, Harris, *From Inuit to Implementation: Omega-3 Fatty Acids Come of Age*, Mayo Clin Proc, June 2000; 75(6):607-14

6. Albert, *Fish Oil – an Appetizing Alternative to Anti-arrhythmic Drugs?* Lancet. 2004 May 1;363 (9419):1412-3; Burr, Fehily, Gilbert, et al., *Effects of Changes in Fat, Fish, and Fibre Intakes on Death and Myocardial Reinfarction: Diet and Reinfarction Trial (DART)*, Lancet. 1989 Sep 30; 2 (8666):757-61; *Dietary Supplementation with n-3 Polyunsaturated Fatty Acids and Vitamin E after Myocardial Infarction: Results of the GISSI-Prevenzione Trial*, Lancet 1999 August 7;354(9177):447-55; Albert, Hennekens, O'Donnell, et al. *Fish Consumption and Risk of Sudden Cardiac Death. JAMA.* 1998 January 7;279(1):23-8.

7. JAMA 1998, Jan 7; 279 (1): 23-8

8. Valenzuela, *Marine Oils: the Health Benefits of N-3 Fatty Acids*, Nutrition. 2000 Jul-Aug;16(7-8):680-4

9. Bloom, Clin. Cardiol. 2004 Sep; 27 (9): 495-500

10. Jahangiri, Leifert, Patten, McMurchie, Mol. Cell Biochem. 2000 Mar; 206 (1-2): 33-41

11. Harris, Curr, *So, Does Taking Fish Oil Prevent AFIB?* Atheroscler. Rep. 2004 Nov; 6 (6): 447-52

12. Crane, Sun, Sun: *The Essential Functions of Coenzyme Q,* Clinical Investigator 71 (suppl 8): S55-S59, 1993; Pepping: *Coenzyme Q,* American Journal of Health-System Pharmacy 56: 519-521, 1999; Rauchova, Drahota, Lenaz, *Function of Coenzyme Q in the Cell: Some Biochemical and Physiological Properties,* Physiol Res. 1995;44(4):209-16

13. Baggio, Gandini, Plancher, Passeri, Carmosino, *Italian Multicenter Study on the Safety and Efficacy of Coenzyme Q10 as Adjunctive Therapy in Heart Failure;* CoQ10 Dug Surveillance Investigators. Mol Aspects Med. 1994;15 Suppl: s287-94

14. Rosenfeldt, Hilton, Pepe, Krum, *Systematic Review of Effect of Coenzyme Q10 in Physical Exercise, Hypertension and Heart Failure,* Biofactors. 2003;18(1-4):91-100

15. *Prevent Heart Attack and Stroke with Potent Enzyme that Dissolves Deadly Blood Clots in Hours,* Health Sciences Institute, March 2002

16. Maruyama, Sumi, *Effect of Natto Diet on Blood Pressure,* JTTAS, 1995

17. These studies involved researchers from Miyazaki Medical College and Kurashiki University of Science and Arts in Japan studied the effects of nattokinase on blood pressure in both animal and human subjects

18. *Prevent Heart Attack and Stroke with Potent Enzyme that Dissolves Deadly Blood Clots in Hours,* Health Sciences Institute, March 2002; Maruyama, Sumi, *Effect of Natto Diet on Blood Pressure.* JTTAS, 1995, Sumi, Hamada, Nakanishi, Hiratani H. Enhancement of the Fibrinolytic Activity in Plasma by Oral Administration of Nattokinase. Acta Haematol 1990;84(3):139-43; Journal of Fibronolysis and Thrombolysis. Abstracts of the Ninth International Congress on Fibrinolysis, Amsterdam, 1988, Vol.2, Sup.1:67; Sumi, Hamada, Tsushima, Mihara, Muraki, *A Novel Fibrinolytic Enzyme (Nattoki nase) in the Vegetable Cheese Natto; a Typical and Popular Soybean Food in the Japanese Diet.* Experientia 1987, Oct 15;43(10):1110-1; Sumi, *Health*

Microbe "Bacillus Natto", Japan Bio Science Laboratory Co. Ltd; Sumi, *Interview With Doctor of Medicine Hiroyuki Sumi.* Japan Bio Science Laboratory Co. Ltd.; Sumi, *Structure and Fibronolytic Properties of Nattokinase*

19. The Guardian, August 13, 2000; New Zealand Medical Journal (Volume 113, Feb 11, 2000; Journal of Agricultural and Food Chemistry, September 2001; Allergy 1999;54;261-265

20. *Evaluation of the Health Aspects of Soy Protein Isolates as Food Ingredients*, prepared for FDA by Life Sciences Research Office, Federation of American Societies for Experimental Biology (9650 Rockville Pike, Bethesda, MD 20014), USA, Contract No. FDA 223-75-2004, 1979; Wall Street Journal, October 27, 1995; Urquhart, *A Health Food Hits Big Time*, Wall Street Journal, August 3, 1999; Natural Medicine News (L & H Vitamins, 32-33 47th Avenue, Long Island City, NY 11101), USA, January/February 2000, p. 8; Harras, *Cancer Rates and Risks*, National Institutes of Health, National Cancer Institute, 1996, 4th edition; Searle, *Chemical Carcinogens, ACS Monograph 173*, American Chemical Society, Washington, DC, 1976; Ishizuki, et al., *The Effects on the Thyroid Gland of Soybeans Administered Experimentally in Healthy Subjects*, Nippon Naibunpi Gakkai Zasshi (1991) 767:622-629; Cassidy, et al., *Biological Effects of a Diet of Soy Protein Rich in Isoflavones on the Menstrual Cycle of Premenopausal Women*, American Journal of Clinical Nutrition (1994) 60:333-340; Setchell, et al., *Isoflavone Content of Infant Formulas and the Metabolic Fate of These Early Phytoestrogens in Early Life*, American Journal of Clinical Nutrition, December 1998 Supplement, 1453S-1461S

21. See also *"Soy: Is it Healthy or is it Harmful?* Dr. Joseph Mercola with Rachael Droege, Jan 21, 2004

22. Personal Nutrition, Fifth Edition, Boyle and Anderson, 2004 Wadsworth

23. Baroody, *Alkalinize or Die*, California: Portal Books, 1995; Haas, *Staying-Healthy with Nutrition – The Complete Guide to Diet & Nutritional Medicine*, Berkeley, California: Celestial Arts, 1992; p. 22; Rona and Martin, *Return to the Joy of Health*, Vancouver: Alive Books, 1995

24. 24. *2004 Kidney function indicates HF prognosis*, Am J Med 2004; 116: 466-473 *2004 Superior protection against MI remodeling with ARBs*, Hypertension 2004; 43: 1-7

25. Boyle and Anderson, *Personal Nutrition*, Wadsworth 2004

26. Enig and Fallon, *The Truth About Saturated Fats – Part I*, Nexus, August 25, 2002. Fallon, *Nourishing Traditions: The Cookbook that Challenges Politically Correct Nutrition and the Diet Dictocrats*

27. Revealing Trans Fats, FDA Consumer Magazine, September/October 2003 Issue

28. Knopp and Retzlaff, *Saturated Fat Prevents Coronary Artery Disease? An American Paradox*, American Journal of Clinical Nutrition, Vol. 80, No. 5, 1102-1103, November 2004

29. Maron, Lu, Cai, et al., *Cholesterol-lowering Effect of a Theaflavin-enriched Green Tea Extract: a Randomized Controlled Trial*, Arch Intern Med. 2003 Jun 23;163(12):1448-53; Willcox, Catignani, Lazarus, *Tomatoes and Cardiovascular Health*, Crit Rev Food Sci Nutr. 2003;43(1):1-18; Devaraj, Vega-Lopez, Kaul, Schonlau, Rohdewald, Jialal, *Supplementation with a Pine Bark Extract Rich in Polyphenols Increases Plasma Antioxidant Capacity and Alters the Plasma Lipoprotein Profile*, Lipids. 2002 Oct;37(10):931-4

30. Berkson, *The Alpha Lipoic Acid Breakthrough*, Three Rivers Press, 1998; Challem, *Quite Possibly the "Universal" Antioxidant*, The Nutrition Reporter, July 1996

31. Cooney, et al., *Gamma Tocopherol Detoxification of Nitrogen Dioxide: Superiority to Alpha Tocopherol*. Proc Natl Acad Sci U S A 1993 Mar 1;90(5):1771-5; Christen, et al., *Gamma Tocopherol Traps Mutagenic Electrophiles Such as NO(X) and Complements Alpha Tocopherol: Physiological Implications*. Proc Natl Acad Sci U S A 1997 Apr 1;94(7):3217-22; Packer, et al., *Molecular Aspects of Alpha Tocotrienol Antioxidant Action and Cell Signalling*, J Nutr 2001 Feb;131(2):369S-73S; Serbinova, et al., *Free Radical Recycling and Intramembrane Mobility in the Antioxidant Properties of Alpha Tocopherol and Alpha Tocotrienol*, Free Radic Biol Med 1991;10(5):263-75

32. Journal of the American College of Nutrition, Dec. 1998, 17(6):601-8); Am. J. Clin. Nutr., (United States), Jan. 1999, 69(1):30-42)

33. Kris-Etherton, Harris, Appel, *Fish Consumption, Fish Oil, Omega-3 Fatty Acids, and Cardiovascular Disease*, Circulation 2002;106:2747.

34. Kennedy, *Strengthen Your Heart: the Herb Arjuna Holds Promise for Those with Cardiovascular Disease – Herb Brief,* Natural Health, Oct-Nov 2002

35. Sabaté, Haddad, Tanzman, Jambazian, and Rajaram, *Research Organization: Loma Linda University Study Title: Serum Lipid Response to the Graduated Enrichment of a Step 1 Diet with Almonds: a Randomized Feeding Trial,* American Journal of Clinical Nutrition, Vol. 77, No. 6, 1379-1384, June 2003

36. Mas, et al., Effects of Policosanol in Patients with Type II Hypercholetse-rolemia and Additional Coronary Risk Factors, Clin Pharmacol Ther 65:439-47 1999; Noa, et al, Effect of Policosanol on Lipofundin-induced Atherosclerotic Lesions in Rats J Pharm Pharmacol 47:289-91 1995; Arru-zazabala, et al., *Protective Effect of Policosanol on Atherosclerotic Lesions in Rabbits with Exogenous Hypercholesterolemia,* Braz J Med Biol Res 33:835-40 2000

37. Menendez R, et al., *Oral Administration of Policosanol Inhibits in Vitro Copper Ion-induced Rat Lipoprotein Peroxidation,* Physiol Behav 67:1-7 1999

38. Arruzazabala, et al., *Comparative Study of Policosanol, Aspirin and the Combination Therapy Policosanol-aspirin on Platelet Aggregation in Healthy Volunteers,* Pharmacol Res 36:293-7 1997; Stusser, et al., *Long-term Therapy with Policosanol Improves Treadmill Exercise-ECG Testing Performance of Coronary Heart Disease Patients,* Int J Clin Pharmacol Ther 36:469-73 1998

39. Tadolini, et al. *Resveratrol Inhibition of Lipid Peroxidation,* Free Radic. Res. 2000;33:105-14

40. Simonini, et al., *Emerging Potentials for an Antioxidant Therapy as a New Approach to the Treatment of Systemic Sclerosis.* Toxicology 2000;155:1-15

41. Zou, et al. *Effect of Red Wine and Wine Polyphenol Resveratrol on Endothelial Function in Hypercholesterolemic Rabbits,* Int. J. Mol. Med. 2003;11:317-20

42. Zbikowska, et al., *Antioxidants with Carcinostatic Activity (Resveratrol, Vitamin E and Selenium) in Modulation of Blood Platelet Adhesion,* J. Physiol. Pharmacol. 2000;51:513-20

43. Montalescot, Ankri, Chadefaux-Vekemans, et al., *Plasma Homocysteine and the Extent of Atherosclerosis in Patients with Coronary Artery Disease*, Int J Cardiol. 1997 Aug 8;60(3):295-300; Stampfer, Malinow, Willett, et al., *A Prospective Study of Plasma Homocysteine and Risk of Myocardial Infarction in US Physicians*, JAMA. 1992 Aug 19;268(7):877-81; Verhoef, Stampfer, Buring, et al., *Homocysteine Metabolism and Risk of Myocardial Infarction: Relation with Vitamins B6, B12, and Folate*, Am J Epidemiol. 1996 May 1;143(9):845-59; Robinson, Mayer, Miller, et al. Hyperhomocysteinemia and Low Pyridoxal Phosphate: Common and Independent Reversible Risk Factors for Coronary Artery Disease, Circulation. 1995 Nov 15;92(10):2825-30; Arnesen, Refsum, Bonaa, Ueland, Forde, Nordrehaug, *Serum Total Homocysteine and Coronary Heart Disease*, Int J Epidemiol. 1995 Aug;24(4):704-9; Pasceri, Willerson, Yeh, *Direct Proinflammatory Effect of C-reactive Protein on Human Endothelial Cells*, Circulation. 2000 Oct 31;102(18):2165-8; Ridker, Stampfer, Rifai, *Novel Risk Factors for Systemic Atherosclerosis: a Comparison of C-reactive Protein, Fibrinogen, Homocysteine, Lipoprotein(a), and Standard Cholesterol Screening as Predictors of Peripheral Arterial Disease*, JAMA. 2001 May 16;285(19):2481-5

44. Cohen, *Magnesium in Hypertension Prevention and Control*, Life Extension Magazine September 2004; Other studies of magnesium can be found in MEDLINE (www.pubmed.org), the National Institutes of Health's vast collection of medical journal articles

45. Rude, *Magnesium Deficiency: a Cause of Heterogeneous Disease in Humans*, J Bone Miner Res. 1998 Apr;13(4):749-58; Cohen, *High-dose Oral Magnesium in the Treatment of Chronic, Intractable Erythromelalgia*, Ann Pharmacother. 2002 Feb;36(2):255-60

46. Iseri, French, *Magnesium: Nature's Physiologic Calcium Blocker*, Am Heart J. 1984 Jul;108(1):18893; Leppert, Myrdal, Hedner, Edvinsson, Tracz, Ringqvist, *Effect of Magnesium Sulfate Infusion on Circulating Levels of Noradrenaline and Neuropeptide-Y-like Immunoreactivity in Patients with Primary Raynaud's Phenomenon*, Angiology. 1994 Jul;45(7):637-45

47. Am J Clin Nutr. 1991 Apr;53(4 Suppl):1027S-1030S

48. Free Radic Biol Med. 1991;10(5):263-75

49. Stocher, *Antioxidant Functions of Vitamin E – Session II*, New York Academy of Science Conference; Gieseg, *Reducing Free Radicals – A Dietary Revolution*, New Zealand Science Monthly, (1999) July, 6-8

50. Kumar, Das, *Are Free Radicals Involved in the Pathology of Human Essential Hypertension?* Free Rad Res Commun 1993; 19(1): 59-66

51. Newez et al., *Effect of Gamma Tocotrienol on Blood Pressure, Lipid Peroxidation and Total Antioxidant Status in Spontaneously Hypertensive Rats (SHR)*, Clin Exp Hyperten 1999; 21(8): 1297-1313

52. Salonen, et al., *Blood Pressure, Dietary Fats, and Antioxidants*, Am Jour Clin Nutr 1988; 48: 1226-32; Enstrom, Kanim, Klein, *Vitamin C Intake and Mortality Among a Sample of the United States Population,* Epidemiology 1992; 3: 194-202; Duffy et al., *Treatment of Hypertension with Ascorbic Acid,* Lancet 1999; 354(9195): 355-64; Taddei et al., *Vitamin C Improves Endothelium-dependent Vasodilation by Restoring Nitric Oxide Activity in Essential Hypertension.* Circulation 1998; 97: 2222-29

53. Medical Research News, Wednesday, July 7, 2004, citing researchers at Wake Forest University Baptist Medical Center

54. September 2004 issue of *Life Sciences*; Research presented at the 6th Annual Conference on Arteriosclerosis, Thrombosis and Vascular Biology held by the American Heart Association April 29, 2005 in Washington, D.C.; New Research Supports Garlic's Role in Arresting and Reversing Arteriosclerosis, American Botanical Council; www.herbalgram.org, the e-newsletter of the American Botanical Council, April 29, 2005; Siegel, Michel, Ploch, Rodriguez, Malmsten, *Inhibition of Arteriosclerotic Plaque Development by Garlic*, Wien Med Wochenschr, 2004 Nov;154(21-22):515-22; Durak, Aytac, Atmaca, Devrim, Avci, Erol, Oral, *Effects of Garlic Extract Consumption on Plasma and Erythrocyte Antioxidant Parameters in Atherosclerotic Patients, Life Sci.* 2004 Sep 3;75(16):1959-66

55. Digiesi, et al., *Mechanism of Action of Coenzyme Q10 in Essential Hypertension*, Curr Ther Res 1992; 51: 668-72; Langsjoen, et al., *Treatment of Essential Hypertension with Coenzyme Q10*, Mol Aspects Med 1994; 15(supp): 265S-72S; Singh, *Effects of Hydrosoluble Coenzyme Q10 on Blood Pressures and Insulin Resistance in Hypertensive Patients with Coronary Artery Disease*, Jour Hum Hyperten 1999; 13: 203-208; Digiesi, Cantini, Brodbeck, *Effect*

of Coenzyme Q10 on Essential Arterial Hypertension, Curr Ther Res 1990; 47; 841-45

56. Aviram, Dornfeld, *Pomegranate Juice Consumption Inhibits Serum Angio-tensin Converting Enzyme Activity and Reduces Systolic Blood Pressure*, Athero-sclerosis. 2001 Sep;158(1):195-8

57. Aviram, Rosenblat, Gaitini, et al., *Pomegranate Juice Consumption for 3 years by Patients with Carotid Artery Stenosis Reduces Common Carotid Intima-media thickness, Blood Pressure and LDL Oxidation*, Clin Nutr. 2004 Jun;23(3):423-33

58. Yang, Lu, Wu, Chang, *The Protective Effect of Habital Tea Consumption on Hypertension*, Arch Intern Med. 2004 Jul 26; 164(14):1534-40

59. *Food and Drug Administration "Final Rule "for Sucralose*, 21 CFR Part 172, Docket No. 87F-0086; Hunter, *Sucralose*, Consumers' Research Magazine, Oct 90, Vol. 73 Issue 10, p8, 2p; *Q&A: Is newly FDA approved sweetener sucralose good for you?* Executive Health's Good Health Report, Nov 98, Vol. 35 Issue 2, p6, 1p, 1c; *Sucralose – a New Artificial Sweetener*, Medical Letter on Drugs & Therapeutics, 07/03/98, Vol. 40, Issue 1030, p67, 2p

60. www.mercola.com

61. Fujimaki 1992, John 1994, Liu 1993, Main 1983; Molhave 1986, National Research Council 1981; Shaham 1996; Srivastava 1992; Vojdani 1992; Wantke 1996

About the Author

I have known and worked with Stuart B. Kalb for over 11 years. Outside of having a keen legal mind, he has a penchant for learning about how to keep oneself in top physical condition and providing practical, common sense solutions for a myriad of health issues. He is a lawyer and yes, he has decided to write a book about a very defined, very specialized health-related issue. There is simply not much written on the subject matter from the standpoint of preventing and alleviating the symptoms of benign heartbeat irregularities. Most readers would question why or how a former U.S. Treasury Department trial lawyer and healthcare lawyer and current transactional estate and elder law attorney can write a book about heart health issues, which are normally considered to be "foreign waters" and otherwise off limits from a professional standpoint. However, having thousands of estate planning clients (many of which have died and all of which will eventually die) leaves plenty of opportunity to evaluate how they lived, why they die and how things may have been different. He has seen hundreds of his clients' families devastated by healthcare costs later in life that the families were never prepared for.

Actually, most of his family, friends, colleagues and even clients, know full well that this arena has been both his passion and his avocation for over two decades. He has studied and analyzed scores of technical papers and reports on all kinds of health-related issues. He has provided a wealth of advice on "natural" non-drug related ideas to lower blood pressure and cholesterol, increase energy, and substantially reduce the risk of having heart disease. He is 56 years of age, but most people are in a complete state of shock when they hear his age and see his face and build. He has the looks of a 45 year old and the physical conditioning better than most men half his age. When time permits he is active in tennis, golf, racquetball, boating, skiing (snow and water), football, softball, table tennis, billiards and more. He is married (22 years) and has two grown children.

He has lectured on the proper foods and supplements to eat and which ones that you absolutely must avoid at all cost. His "disciples" swear by his recommendations and love his no nonsense, practical and easy to understand approach to things that are typically too complicated to understand. The book reflects this style.

But, with all that, he has one problem...he has been the victim of irregular heartbeats despite his otherwise near perfect health. Frustrated with the sheer inadequacies of the state of traditional medicine in addressing this most perplexing issue of heart health, Mr. Kalb set out on a quest to find an answer to the question of irregular heartbeats in otherwise healthy individuals and how to demonstrably reduce or even eliminate its symptoms, and investigate many easy, inexpensive, natural and safe ways to keep the entire cardiovascular system running smoothly without overly expensive and burdensome prescription drugs. This quest has taken over 15 years now and has culminated in this book.

His legal background has obviously given him the training and experience to take complicated subject matter and explain it to lay people so that they can understand it. As a lawyer, he has a different frame of reference: he does not trust the mammoth drug companies who, with their exorbitantly high drug prices and, in his opinion, their effective control of the FDA, are fueled by the profit motive, not patient safety. He is neither paid financial incentives by drug companies to recommend their products, nor is he given all expense paid trips to medical conferences around the globe to learn about promoting their products. He also does not trust the food distribution companies because their focus is on profits for the shareholders rather than nutrition for the consumers.

A lawyer has a different frame of reference with respect to a particular medical issue than the traditional medical community's approach toward such issue. His focus is more on notions of caution, the protection of one's rights, harm, damages and prevention. His perspective on heart health will give you a whole new, refreshing outlook on keeping the most important organ in your body in excellent working order.

Laurie S. Abelbeck, J. D., partner and friend of Stuart B. Kalb

Index

A

Ablation 4, 29, 30, 31

Abnormal Heart Rhythms 49, 51

ACE 53, 54, 162, 163

ACE inhibitors 53, 54, 162, 163

Acrylamide 123

Actiase 57

ADHD 60, 178

Adrenaline 24, 34, 35, 62, 68, 75, 76, 77, 79, 161, 178

Adrenergic Receptors 161, 162

AFIB 14, 15, 17, 18, 20, 21, 22, 23, 24, 25, 26, 27, 28, 29, 30, 31, 32, 33, 34, 39, 42, 49, 51, 61, 66, 68, 72, 81, 82, 85, 90, 142, 162, 165, 166, 190, 194

ALA 43, 140, 142

Aldosterone 163

Allicin 142, 174

Alpha Blockers 4, 162

Alpha-linolenic acid 43

Alpha-lipoic acid 140

Alpha-tocopherol 140, 170

Alternative Remedies xvii, xix

Alzheimer's Disease 36, 109, 178, 191

Amalgam Fillings 37, 80

Ambien 72

Amino Acids 54, 84, 172, 173, 174, 184

Amiodarone 19, 26

Amlo-dipine 169

Angina xviii, 51, 52, 61, 75, 101, 143, 162

Angiotensin Converting Enzyme 54, 163, 200

Angiotensin I 54, 163

Angiotensin II 54, 163

Angiotensin-converting Enzyme Inhibitors 162

Anti-arrhythmia Drugs 4, 30, 32

Anti-hypertensive Drug 175

Antioxidants 74, 75, 89, 108, 109, 111, 115, 125, 138, 139, 140, 146, 171, 197, 199

Anti-platelet drug 28

Anxiety xx, 10, 14, 24, 32, 34, 49, 71, 75, 76, 161

Aorta 7, 9, 142, 151

Apolipoprotein A 130

Apolipoprotein B 131, 153

Apoprotein B 131

Apoproteins 130

Arachidonic acid 41

Arginine 172, 173

Arjuna 143, 197

Arrhythmia 4, 9, 11, 13, 14, 15, 16, 17, 18, 19, 20, 23, 29, 30, 31, 32, 33, 38, 39, 40, 42, 49, 50, 51, 82, 90, 93, 154, 189

Arsenic 64, 65

Arteries 7, 35, 52, 53, 57, 61, 68, 75, 84, 98, 99, 100, 101, 102, 103, 108, 109, 112, 113, 118, 121, 122, 131, 133, 140, 142, 144, 146, 147, 148, 150, 151, 154, 157, 158, 159, 160, 161, 162, 163, 175, 186, 189

Arterioles 161, 162, 163, 169

Arthritis xv, 43, 54, 74, 109, 178

Aspirin 28, 52, 53, 61, 145, 197

Astaxanthin 47

Asthma 34, 60, 178

Atherogenic 117

Atherosclerosis 53, 84, 98, 99, 100, 101, 130, 133, 140, 159, 176, 179, 198, 200

978-0-595-3645(
0-595-36450-(

Made in the USA
Charleston, SC
17 December 2009